Praise for *The Heart Of The Doula*

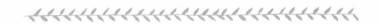

"Amy Gilliland is uniquely qualified to trace, explore, analyze, evaluate, and clarify the role of the doula in maternity care today... Amy's skill in deconstructing the issues and analyzing the many opinions and interpretations that were expressed by interviewees helps readers broaden their thinking... this work provides clarity and guidance on what doulas really do and really should do!

All doulas will benefit from this book. I can even picture it being used as a discussion guide for groups."

Penny Simkin, PT, CD(DONA)
Co-Founder of DONA International and their first Birth Doula Trainer
Certified Childbirth Educator, Author, Researcher

"Amy's essays left me with a warm, tender, deep, and purposeful feeling – the kind of renewal every doula (and every human) needs once in a while...Her illustration of the complexity and variety of doula work is astounding, and she shows deep understanding of the way doula skills develop and complement existing supports."

Molly Mendota, AdvCD/BDT(DONA)
DONA International Birth Doula Trainer, *Health Connect One* Birth Equity Leadership Faculty

"This is a great book for student doulas, new doulas, and those already in the field that can help them understand some of the professional boundaries that they will encounter as we work to define what it really means to do our job...I would love to recommend this to my own students."

Rachel Leavitt, RN, BSN, CD, New Beginnings Doula Trainings

"I'm reading it with lots of smiles and nods and some tears, as your words speak the truth about this amazing calling/career/vocation. I'm so glad you've written this and I can't wait to add it to my Steps for Success for new doulas, and to recommend it as a keeper for their entire journey!"

Ana M. Hill, IBCLC, CLD, CLE, CCCE, Rocky Mountain Doula Training

"*The Heart of a Doula* should be a prerequisite for all doula training programs. Amy accurately captures the intricacies and nuances of what it means to be a doula and her insights will help the reader to not only be a better doula but a better human as well...It is a must read for new and seasoned doulas alike."

Caity Ann Mehl, Columbus Birth & Parenting
Birth/Postpartum Doula Trainer (DONA International & ProDoula, retired)

"She has answered the questions the majority of new doulas have on their minds. This book can serve the purpose of an experienced mentor, helping doulas to think more critically and expansively about the nuances of this privileged role they are fulfilling, thereby bolstering their self-confidence...Most of all, I felt that I had just had a very in-depth conversation with a wise and trusted colleague."

Sunday Tortelli, LCCE, AdvCD/BDT(DONA), DONA International Birth Doula Trainer

"Being a doula can in some ways be a lonely job...when we can, doulas gravitate towards each other to talk shop, compare notes, share what we've learned, and process the good, the bad, and the ugly about what we have experienced supporting others in labor...Amy embodies that cooperative spirit with this new work, a gift to the doula community."

Julie Brill, IBCLC, CLD, CCCE, CAPPA Labor Doula Faculty
Author, *Round the Circle: Doulas Share Their Experiences*

The Heart

OF THE

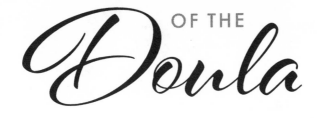

Doula

Essentials for Practice and Life

AMY L. GILLILAND

Ph.D., BDT(DONA), CSE (AASECT)

TABLE OF CONTENTS

Introduction

Being a birth doula is one of the most complex tasks on the planet. Being successful requires a high degree of emotional intelligence plus self awareness, self control, physical ability, clear psychological boundaries, and professional ethics. Also needed are the ability to communicate effectively and negotiate conflict with clients and careproviders of all kinds. None of these things are skills that can be covered thoroughly in a birth doula training workshop. Doulas need a guide to help figure out how to navigate the medical system and make ethical choices when they're in the midst of a complex problem.

In their workshops, trainers concentrate on passing along childbirth knowledge, physical support skills, and their own hard earned wisdom. They want the emotional guidance given to trainees to stay with them as they continue on their doula journey. This book reinforces the important principles that trainers try to impart in the short time they have with our participants. But it also goes further, showing how you as a doula can truly transform another person's life, changing it for the better.

Doulas are powerful. With our guidance, our clients become more empowered versions of themselves. They are able to grow and become more like the person they want to be. That's part of being of service to another human being – we're there to assist and to guide after *they* have chosen the destination. In this same way, I hope this book will also help you to become the heart-centered doula that you want to be. While the written voice is mine, the wisdom is culled from over sixty doulas that I formally interviewed and the thousands who I have conversed with in my three decades of doulaing. The research is explained thoroughly in *About The Study*.

I truly believe that we serve best when we observe and get out of our client's way. We lead by following. We show up for them in a way no one else can. We don't leave. We don't have an agenda or preference. Our mantras are "It's not my birth", and "It's not my baby." We maintain an aura of detachment from their choices, but this also comes at a personal cost.

A doula's life is like no other. Our whole goal is to not be in control! We exist in the moment, mindful, in a breath. That's hard work. Being in control, multi-tasking, taking charge – those are all behaviors that get repeatedly rewarded in modern society. Doula work is the antithesis of constant hurrying and seeking control, so we don't get recognized for the supportive, nurturing skills we've been challenged to develop.

Caring skills are often dismissed as something anyone could do because most humans have the capacity to care. But that doesn't mean they develop their brains to really practice the art of caring well for others. We know that repeated practice of a skill causes growth in parts of the brain related to that skill. Based on that, I hypothesize that the brains of experienced birth doulas are different from people who don't practice these same skills. By supporting people at bedside during their births, our amygdalae become highly attuned to their biobehavioral cues, and are repeatedly bathed in oxytocin stimulating environments for hours and days at a time. I'm willing to bet large sums of money that a magnetic resonance imaging (MRI) study of doulas who'd attended over a hundred births would show more highly developed brain structures used to recognize interpersonal cues, interpret the emotional content of other's behaviors, and positively influence social harmony. (To read more, please see Carter, 2017.)

This book addresses a wide range of issues where doulas may need to make decisions. Some of those decisions can be very challenging to make. We find ourselves wondering, "What is the right thing to do? What factors do I need to consider? Whose perspectives might I be missing? If there is a conflict, whose values do I honor?" Sometimes there is no right answer, there's just a choice to be made and you will need to consider multiple points of view. This book offers you those perspectives, expanding around your own individual dilemma so that you can see what other considerations need to be taken into account.

Doulas are often making value-laden decisions. "Do we put the client's needs *always* first or do we need to consider how our actions will reflect on other doulas? Do you honor the intentions laid out in the birth plan or do you respect the choices that are now being made in labor? When a client asks about your births, is that what they really want to know? How do you negotiate working with all the different kinds of nurses, midwives, and physicians that you'll encounter? How do you become a part of a support team when you've never even met your teammates before?"

If the Doula Disappeared... outlines the invisible actions that birth doulas do. We make a huge difference in our clients' birth experiences but rarely get noticed. *Are There Enough Clients For All Of Us?*, *Why It's A Calling*, and *Another Reason Birth Is Sacred* expressed the core beliefs held by many doulas in the study. I found that having these beliefs enabled them to successfully traverse the internal territory of doulaing as well as getting along with their peers.

The Scope of Practice essays on *The Essential (Oil) Dilemma* and *What It Means To Be A Professional Birth Doula* challenge some of the ways people interpret doula work and our purpose. Are we an 'intervention' or a core piece of the design of labor process that has finally been recognized? The voice in those two essays is primarily mine, but the questions each essay poses, well, you will have to answer them for yourself.

Participant voices in my study were loud and clear about whose needs should take priority in the doula-client relationship and how to integrate that priority into practice. *Understanding Why Mothers Choose A Particular Doula* explains that these choices have little to do to with anything the doula can control. This may be frustrating and freeing at the same time.

The next four selections: *Why Not To Share Your Birth Story*, *Showing Up*, *The Art of Labor Sitting*, and *Why You Should Keep Your Hands To Yourself* focus on what it means to deeply support someone else and put their interests first - before our own needs. We think about those things philosophically but these essays explain how you enact this knowledge in real life.

Being Who She Needs You To Be sounds wonderful, until what your client needs you to be is the scapegoat, or the person who didn't do their job right – even when you had no control over the situation. Though these experiences are uncommon, when they happen it can feel frustrating, troubling and sometimes demeaning. But it happens often enough that we need to recognize it is real life for doulas. The second of these essays will help to understand why clients behave this way, and why discussing these situations with other doulas can be very helpful.

The next five essays are about working alongside medical professionals and building solid relationships whenever you can. This is the area that vexes most doulas and where they want the most guidance. This section helps people to understand the various perspectives medical people have and how that influences their behavior. Whether we like it or not, thriving at hospital births is necessary for doulas' continued success – both individually and as a social movement.

Lastly, *Powerful Prenatal Relationships* pulls it all together. The eleven core tenets of my Doulaing The Doula™ philosophy are shared here. When you put them all together, your inner work on yourself and your approach to clients, you will truly be able to have powerful transformative relationships that create lasting positive change in their lives.

Doula work is a unique profession. We deal with the intangible and the unexplainable. We stand in our own strength letting things be the way they are without trying to fix them or pretty them up. We are deeply intimate during a vulnerable transition in people's lives. Then we move away, having helped them to find strength and abilities they didn't know they possessed. Our services are needed and valuable. When we hold this as truth inside ourselves, we know who we are. That transforms everybody.

References:

Carter, S. S. (2017). The Role of Oxytocin and Vasopressin In Attachment. *Psychodynamic Psychiatry, 45*(4), 499-518.

Roth, L., Henley, M., Seacrist, M., & Morton, C. (2016). North American Nurses' and Doulas' Views of Each Other. *JOGNN-Journal of Obstetric Gynecologic and Neonatal Nursing, 45*, 790-800.

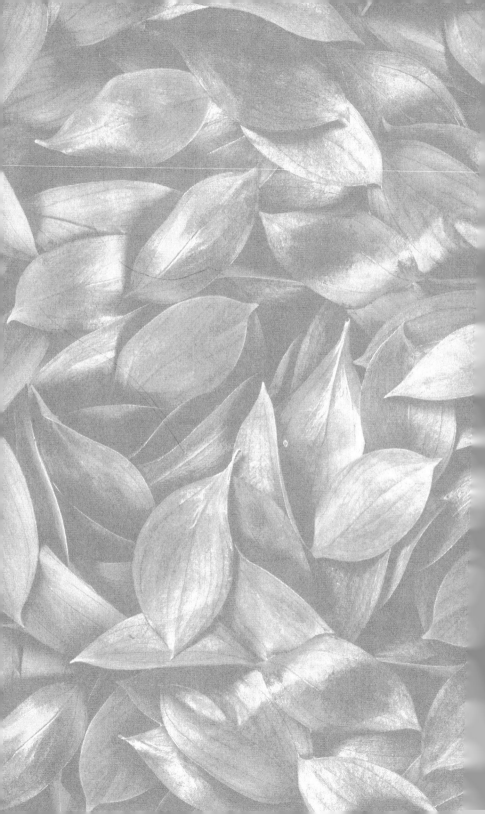

About The Study

When I began graduate school I had no intention of studying doulas. Doulaing was something I did, a doula was something I was, and now I wanted to be more. I wanted to return to the life I'd had before I had children, before motherhood and empowerment through pregnancy and childbirth had become my life's work. I didn't want to leave birth work behind, but I was ready for Something Else.

I leapt into the mental discipline of qualitative research – of analyzing people's words and nuances to see the commonalities between their experiences. One of my advisors, the late Betty Black, told me to study what I knew - doulas, especially because very few studies had been done about what doulas did, how they thought, or how they operated in the world. That was in 2002 and I've been studying birth doulas ever since. It took ten years to earn my Master's of Science and my Doctorate degrees from one of the most highly regarded social science research programs in the country. My thesis and dissertation combined totaled over 900 pages. Eighty to two hundred pages was a more typical length in my field, but I just could not stop – there was too much wisdom in these doulas' words.

My work has been published in the peer reviewed journals *JOGNN – Journal of Obstetrical, Gynecological, and Neonatal Nursing*; *Midwifery*; *Sexuality & Culture*; the *Wisconsin Medical Journal* and the *Journal of Perinatal Education*. My work has also been published in the first academic book on doula support, *Intimate Labour: Birth, Bodies, and Boundaries*; and the advice book for new doulas, *Round The Circle*. The reason that I started my blog, *Doulaing The Doula*, in 2013 was primarily to disseminate my research findings that were relevant to doula practice. The essays in this book address the categories of data that didn't fit neatly into an article for a peer reviewed journal.

What research method did you use to obtain and analyze your data? How did you get the sample of doulas?

I interviewed doulas in waves, which was appropriate for the research method I was using called "grounded theory". With grounded theory, the researcher does some interviews, then analyzes them for commonalities, then does some more interviews to expand on the information they have already gathered. The goal is to keep pushing the boundaries of the sample by including participants who have different backgrounds, experiences, or perspectives. When a perspective or concept doesn't fit with the ideas found earlier, a researcher is forced to change their ideas to include the new information ("negative case analysis"). Only by pushing for diversity is it possible to find the best explanation or answers to the "why" and "how" questions that qualitative research can answer. When the researcher keeps interviewing more diverse participants or circumstances but stops getting new concepts, the study has reached "saturation". That's when it is time to stop collecting data and analyze it more deeply. At this stage, the answers are in there.

In 2002 and 2003, I interviewed 28 doulas from ten different states in the U.S. and two Canadian provinces. To be included in the study participants had to have attended at least 25 births, speak English fluently and not use any clinical skills (e.g. listening to fetal heart tones, taking blood pressure readings, doing vaginal exams to measure cervical dilation) as a doula or in any other job role. All the doulas identified as cisgendered women.

These doulas practiced in large cities, small cities, and rural areas. Two worked for hospital doula programs and twenty-six had their own independent practices. They had attended 25 to 500 births apiece. Participants came from various economic classes and religious faiths, and ranged in age from 28 to 60. About 80% were White, which was typical of doulas in that time period (Lantz & Low, 2005). They had received their training from DONA, CAPPA, ICEA or CBI (Childbirth International); about half were certified.

Then I interviewed parents who had hired their own doulas (not the study participants), and did several rounds of analysis. I had several theories by then, but I wasn't satisfied. I needed a more diverse group of doulas.

I set my sights on interviewing doulas who worked for hospitals as well as parents who had received their services. I'm indebted to Cindy Kerbs, RN, the director of the *Lexington Medical Center Doula Program* in Columbia, South Carolina, for helping me to gain access to their doulas and patients. In 2005, I made three trips to Columbia and interviewed six staff doulas, twelve couples, four mothers, and seven nurses about their experiences with birth doula support.

Then I took a five year break from interviews to analyze the data, complete my dissertation and achieve my doctorate in 2010. After graduating, I interviewed another ten doulas who worked for three different hospital based programs in Minneapolis. I needed the additional data to complete my study on hospital based doulas and their dilemmas.

Do you think the sample is representative of the birth doula population?

Yes. I think that for the time it was done, this sample was representative of the birth doula population. My sample matched the characteristics in the only survey study ever done of doulas at that point, published in 2005 (Lantz & Low). This book, published in 2018, is based on interviews done over an eight year period with forty-four doulas who were diverse in region, population they serve, facilities they work in, economic status, religion, race and ethnicity, age, marital status, and birth responsibilities. "Saturation" was reached and then tested for again. It also includes interviews with parents.

You also had parents in your sample. Is that unusual?

Doulaing is about relationship. You can't doula in a room all by yourself. It made sense to me to examine the relationship. I wanted to figure out how doulas acted out the behaviors of relating in a doulaing way with parents. To do that effectively, I'd need to talk to both sets of informants – the people doing the doulaing as well as the people receiving it. This is unique as I haven't seen any other explanatory study like this on the topic. Maybe that's why it's so deep and powerful.

First I interviewed ten mothers from three Midwestern states in the U.S. who lived in cities and rural areas, and ranged in age from 25 to 38 years old. Nine were married; two were multiparas. Fathers attended all of the births. These parents had hired their doula and worked with her during pregnancy and postpartum. Most took a childbirth class.

My criteria for any parents to be included in the study sample were that the mothers needed to be over 18 years old, speak English fluently, have had uncomplicated pregnancies with no life threatening complications during the labor, and had their first or second live birth. An additional support person close to the birthing mother had to have been present the entire time the doula was there. In each case doula support had been continuous, the doula had used no clinical skills, the infant had spent no time in the NICU, and if a cesarean birth occurred, it had not been due to a medical emergency.

When I got to Columbia, South Carolina, I was thrilled. Many of the parents I interviewed didn't even know what a doula was when they arrived in labor at Lexington Medical Center. The admitting nurse offered them the doula's services and assured the parents they could send the doula away if they didn't like her. Other parents had chosen Lexington Medical Center because they wanted a doula and couldn't afford to hire one. These parents were very diverse in age, race, economic means, education, urban or rural background, number of children, type of birth they wanted (and got), and relationship status. In this group some of the women were single or were accompanied by a person other than their partner or father of the baby.

You mentioned that you focused on the relationship between doulas and parents. Can you explain more about what that means and how that makes this study special?

Most studies focus on the behavior of a *group* of people or a *type* of individual. It's really hard to get at the nuances of a relationship using those approaches. My research training is in Human Development and Family Studies. Families are all about relationships. Humans don't develop on their own; we develop in relation to other family members, to how we view ourselves, and to our environment. Examining relationships was something I was trained to do, but that didn't make it easy. (This type of research is very different from psychology, which examines the interior life of an individual, and sociology, which is mostly concerned with the behaviors of groups of people.)

After my first three interviews, it quickly became clear that what I had tapped into was related to attachment and parent-infant relationships. I kept hearing the same language and terms to describe mother-doula and parent-infant connections. I knew then that looking at relationships and not characteristics of the individual people would to lead me to answers about what doulas do, how they think, and how they interacted with parents and professionals to produce these positive effects on relationships. As of this writing, I don't know of any one else who has done that. But it's the wisdom of all these doulas and the parents who received their care that gives us this book.

How did you analyze the data?

First I transcribed the recorded interviews into written copy. I did this myself for the first ten, and then listened to the recording to check and make notes once I hired a professional transcriber. I analyzed each person's interview line by line, and sentence by sentence, making notes in the margins. About half the doula interviews were over thirty pages long, but parent interviews were usually about 18 pages. I identified concepts in each line and then eventually grouped them together from different interviews. Each concept was then defined by how it related to other concepts. In the olden days I used a bulletin board, index cards, and yarn to illustrate their relationships! For my dissertation I was able to use a computer program. However I only used it to catalog the relationships and concepts that I identified in my own head, never to do the analysis.

The idea behind grounded theory is for the researcher to use their own analytical skills and knowledge of the phenomena to break each concept down into its smallest parts. When I was examining an idea, such as "Why Not To Share Your Birth Story", I needed to discern whether there was another core idea nested inside that one. If so, then I needed to break it down even more and identify how that idea influenced or related to doulas sharing their own birth stories. Once all the concepts were broken down into their smallest parts and the relationships to the other concepts were defined, my job as a researcher was to step back, examine my findings from different angles and get a sense of the holistic nature of the phenomena. As I put this all back together again, I saw how those concepts functioned together and influenced one another. I was able to explain the *function* of those ideas as well as the *process* of how they work. That's the hardest part of this project, but something I've been able to do quite effectively in explaining *The Doula Effect*.

Do you think being a doula helped or hurt your research?

It definitely helped 95% of the time! Participants were more willing to open up to me and share more deeply because they understood I would "get it". I was also able to ask more insightful questions. Parents were more willing to be interviewed and to invite me into their homes because I was a doula. One of the concerns about being an insider is that you might assume that you share ideas in common with your informants when you really don't. So I had a sticky note on my tape recorder to remind me to always ask, when a term was used, to ensure that we were defining it the same way.

Having done doula work for almost twenty years gave me an incredible advantage in analyzing the data. I understood what one informant meant when she said, "I lead by following her, and amplifying what her cues are telling me about what she needs." Many times a participant put into words something that I had experienced. This also meant that I didn't get caught up in the surface content, but pushed for deeper meaning, which showed up in the findings.

Where did the titles of your essays or names for these concepts come from?

Most of the titles I use are excerpts from things said by the doulas and parents I interviewed, to describe their experiences. Other titles wouldn't have been potent enough or descriptive enough to convey the participants' meaning. For example, "Showing Up", "Mother's Goals Become Doula's Goals", and "Being Whoever She Needs Me to Be" are ways these doulas described how they decided which support strategies to use. I tried to be as true as I could to their ideas.

Do you consider your research study to exemplify reliability and validity?

Reliability and validity apply to quantitative research, in which researchers gather data to generate a statistical analysis that describes phenomena. One important criteria is for other people to be able to repeat your study – and for the research method to be transparent and meet strict scientific standards. Quantitative research is good for answering the questions, "How many or how often?" It can also provide statistical modeling to see which factors might be the most influential on a particular situation. But it can't identify what those factors are or explain *why* they're important. For that you need qualitative research (like this study), which is judged by separate standards. Instead of statistical reliability and validity, researchers using grounded theory strive for trustworthiness, which is the degree to which the interpretations of the data accurately describe the phenomena under investigation. Trustworthiness has four criteria for judging the soundness of qualitative research: transferability, credibility, confirmability, and dependability.

Transferability estimates the extent to which the results of the inquiry can be generalized to other contexts or settings. Credibility is an appraisal of whether the interpretation of the data is plausible and represents participants' original data accurately. Confirmability signifies the degree to which other researchers could corroborate the findings and interpretations. Dependability refers to the idea that the research study could be repeated, resulting in the same core findings. It also means that the researcher needs to account for changes that occur within the setting, to the researcher, or social influences that might shift the findings. In other words, a world event or personal experience may shift the meaning or interpretation of the data and needs to be accounted for within the analysis.

In my dissertation, which is available on my web site, www.amygilliland.com, there are details about how I fully met each of these criteria. In addition, each of the concepts was confirmed by a meeting of doulas who were not interviewed (focus group) to see if my wording and understanding accurately described their experience.

In conclusion, I am a hundred percent satisfied that the research conclusions and essays included in this book are an accurate representation of birth doula's thoughts, concerns, and philosophies in the first decade of the twenty first century.

The doulas and parents in your sample were interviewed between 2002 and 2010. Has anything changed since then that might influence your findings?

There are definite differences in technology and in obstetrical practice. We've gone from cell phones to smart phones with apps. There are more ways to communicate with people long distance. Most people know what a doula is without lengthy explanations. Doula organizations have gone international. We went from the "Big Five" training organizations (DONA, CAPPA, ALACE, Childbirth International, ICEA) to more than eighty listed on DoulaMatch.net in early 2018. Birth doula support has been recognized as beneficial by the American College of Obstetricians and Gynecologists (ACOG), and people are recommended to stay home in early labor, and eat and drink as they wish. The cesarean birth rate is above 32%. Evidence Based Birth (evidencebasedbirth.com) is now making research conclusions available to everyday people. Even pleasure is part of our conversation about childbirth these days.

Probably the biggest change has been the commodification of labor support: it is now seen as something that is worth paying for. Labor support is now a viable product in the free market; it is recognized as a commodity to be bought or sold. Doulas are part of the labor force and we are respected as a paid paraprofessional in many settings. That's probably the biggest change.

But has the core of doulaing changed? No.

Has the nature of the work – the labor that is actually performed – changed? No.

Have people's needs in labor changed? No.

Has the structure of the relationship between medical care providers and patients been altered? No.

Are there any additional constraints or limitations on the way that doulas practice their craft? No.

Has the system of medical care in the United States changed in a way that affects the way that perinatal care is delivered? No.

Do people still need to be reminded that they have a voice that should be heard? Yes.

So the core tasks of birth doula support, the people who provide it, the people who receive it, and the arena in which support is delivered have not substantially changed. Because of that, this work passes the test of time.

References

Creswell, J. (1998) *Qualitative Inquiry and Research Design: Choosing Among Five Traditions,* Sage Publications, Thousand Oaks.

American College of Obstetrics and Gynecologists. (2017) Approaches to Limit Intervention During Labor and Birth. *Committee Opinion*, Vol. 687 ACOG.

James, K. (2018) Personal communication Re www.doulamatch.net.

Lantz, P.M., Low, L.K., Varkey, S. & Watson, R.L. (2005) Doulas as childbirth paraprofessionals: Results from a national survey. *Womens Health Issues,* **15**(3), 109-116.

Strauss, A. & Corbin, J. (1998) *Basics of Qualitative Research,* Sage Publications, Thousand Oaks, CA.

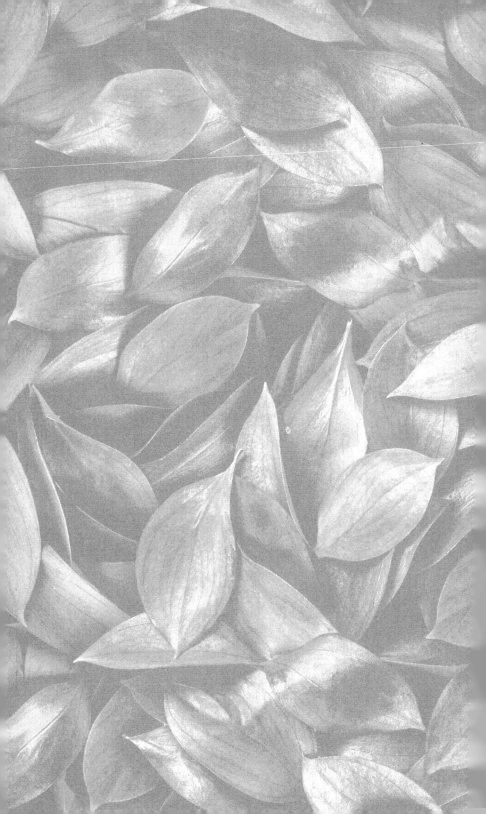

Foundations

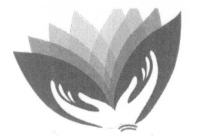

If The Doula Disappeared, No One Would...

Shut the door

Cover every toe with the blanket

Make sure the curtains overlap

Persevere until we find just the right spot

Remind you to ask questions

Repeat what was said to you during a contraction

Move the yukky towels from your sight and smell right away

Shut the door again

Restart the playlist

Work with your nurse, helping him or her to get to know you

Repeat your visualization with each contraction

Be calm

Be the extra pair of hands

Fetch anything you wanted

Anticipate what you need

Keep a catalog in their head of what makes you feel better

Have your comfort and well being as the #1 priority

Make sure your loved ones are informed

Know how to interpret your medical provider's concerns in language a tired laboring brain can understand

Shut the door again

Give your partner a break and remind him or her its okay to eat

Keep the focus on you

Remind you that you are having a baby

Help the nurse

Tape your photos in the room

Understand medical procedures and explain what you might feel in advance

Believe in you and your ability to birth your baby

Remind you that you can say "no" or "not now"

Help you find your voice

Be there with you the whole time

Make sure your partner got to do what he or she wanted to

Shut the door again

Remember to fetch the baby book

Change the room temperature

Recall your deepest birth dreams and help to make them happen

Console you when they don't

Reflect your rhythms

Take detailed notes of what people say and write down what happened

Empower you to advocate for what you want

Try other things first

Disappear when you need privacy

Understand how each pain medication may affect you and your baby

Know your birth memories and satisfaction will affect you the rest of your life

Protect the space

Keep irrelevant activities from distracting you

Offer unconditional support free from future obligations

Be your doula

I've often said that no one notices what the doula does; they only notice if she's not there. The professional doula often works in the background to make things run more smoothly and help people to get along. Of course doulas do more than what is on this list but those activities (i.e. comfort measures, encouragement) can also be done by nurses and loved ones. This list is about what we uniquely bring to the labor room. It is based on my interviews with sixty doulas and parents about their experiences.

Are There Enough Clients For All Of Us?

D o you feel that you are competing with every other doula for clients? *"There's not enough for me and for everyone else. If someone else gets a client, that's one I don't have."* And then you try to work harder to compete and get ahead. (Or you give up.) Fearing there isn't enough to go around means believing in scarcity.

Let's break down that idea – Are There Enough Clients To Go Around?

From a rational perspective, the answer is clearly "yes". According to the Listening To Mothers III survey, 6% of people in the sample had a birth doula but 27% of them wanted one. That's a huge gap between demand and supply. Granted not all of those people may be willing to pay a doula a sustainable fee. But the doula's biggest market is second time parents! They are more aware of the doula's value and will pay money not to repeat their first experience. Unfortunately they did not report on postpartum doulas in the survey, but many people have had postpartum experiences they don't want to repeat either.

From a marketing perspective, the answer is also "yes". By profiling and targeting your ideal client, you learn that the best person for you to work with isn't "everybody who is pregnant". No matter how wonderful you are, you are not everyone's best doula. It really is a select group. When you compare your ideal client to those of other doulas, you realize that you are after different markets. Of course there will be some overlap and not all of your clients will fit the ideal profile, but many will be close to the target. I find that reassuring – we're not all after the same person but different kinds of pregnant people.

From a personal perspective, the answer is always "yes". People choose their doula based on whom they feel safe with in their gut, not on how good your welcome packet looks. (The welcome packet opens the door and introduces you.) We have no control over that decision except to be our authentic selves.

For my nineteen years as a doula trainer, I have been preaching that it never makes sense for doulas to compete with each other, no matter what organization they trained with. There's no economic reason to do that because the market isn't saturated. When one doula gets a client, it generates interest in the market among other potential buyers of our services. The more people we serve, the more interest grows, and more our potential market grows. Every nine months there is a complete turnover. So our best strategy to grow the profession is to support each other while also pursuing our own individual goals. Abundance is out there. The more we work for success together, the more there will be for all of us.

Every doula I have trained understands this. There are plenty of potential clients and the more we work together to educate the public and careproviders, the more paying clients we will all get. The doula leaders in our region (past and present) also reflect this attitude, and because of it we have a more collegial and supportive atmosphere in our state than in many of the places I visit across the U.S.

When we choose scarcity, we choose fear. Fear that there won't be enough. Fear that someone else will get the good stuff first. Fear that if someone else does well, that means we'll do poorly. There isn't enough cake for everyone to have a piece even if we slice it small! Our bodies end up feeling tight and tense and we worry about what we can do to get more and to get it for ourselves.

Rather than thinking "not enough", think "there is enough". It doesn't cost you anything to shift from a mindset of scarcity to one of abundance, except your level of personal responsibility. With a scarcity mindset, all of your problems are "out there". The locus of control is outside of you and thus uncontrollable. But when you believe that abundance exists, your attention becomes focused on how to tap into it. You have an internal locus of control – "*what I do and how I do it influences my circumstances*".

As this process advances, you'll become more optimistic – the best is yet to come! You're more willing to take risks and share your self and resources with colleagues. You can learn from your competitors because you are all in this together. As your relationships with other doulas grow, you can ask for feedback and help without it feeling like a threat. Babies will continue to be conceived and people will keep recognizing that their emotional needs are not being met by current medical systems. That isn't going to change anytime soon.

What About Not Having Enough Time?

My worst tendency towards scarcity is about time. I fear there will never be enough time to get everything done; that I won't achieve my dreams much less what's on my daily 'to do' list. "There just isn't enough time!!" Sound familiar? I'm not competing with other people for time – its not like if I get more someone else gets less. I'm really competing with myself – and I never win.

The funny thing is that it's not true. I do have enough time. Sometimes it takes me until Wednesday to get through Monday's to do list, but it does get done. The small tasks and the big projects do get completed, for the most part. So what's going on here? It's all in my attitude. Being anxious that I don't have enough time doesn't get me more time, nor does it make me more creative or efficient. It just makes me jittery and unpleasant. So, what's my alternative?

I decided to change my thought. "Time expands to meet my needs." Whenever I begin to have the impending feeling of doom – "there will never be enough" – I realize it's all in my head. *Whatever really needs to happen will and I will have enough time to accomplish it.* It's been four months now, and I have accomplished everything I needed to do. Some things got postponed, true, but it was mostly because the time wasn't right – and even I can't do everything at once. In some instances my priorities changed. But what was really different was my compassion for myself and my anxieties.

Our approach to life is up to us. We choose how we want to think about life. I prefer to choose abundance.

Why It's A Calling...

Doula work is hard! It is physically challenging, emotionally draining and requires a personal connection that leaves life long impressions. Doulas sacrifice to be there for their clients. They prioritize other people's birth memories above the needs of their own families. They get paid less than what they are worth – often wages are barely above the poverty line. There is a limit to how many clients one can physically and psychically manage. Yet, this work is something that so many of us cannot imagine *not* doing. It fulfills some part of who we are – it expresses our life essence. To help another person through childbirth – as they are physically going through the process of giving life to another human being – is what we feel we are *called* to do.

A calling is often referred to in religious terms because that is our most familiar cultural reference. But a calling means that there is a purpose within us to connect to others and improve their lives. We want to ensure that another person's journey is eased by our presence. What we give is not only a skill or a service, but the essence of our own humanity. Doulas in my study said it was a passion, a priority, without doulaing they would feel that a part of them was missing.

Ten of the sixty doulas in my study described or mentioned the word "calling". Tracy said, "Being a doula is a part of who you are. You can't try to be a doula…you either have it in you or you don't." Nancy shared, "It's my passion and it tests my compassion. In my real life, I'm a banker! But that's a career and this is a passion." Sadie said, "It was in my heart. For so long before I took my workshop I knew it was in my heart and I've never been happier even though it's been so hard."

The calling of birth doula work often comes at great cost. I'm not talking about the missed birthday parties or band recitals, although those certainly matter. It cost us when we sit holding hands of a woman who is being victimized by her own choices, or who is not respected because she is young, not white, or doesn't speak English. When we SEE that infants are whole human beings with a full consciousness and no one else acts in a way that acknowledges it, it costs us. When we know a physician feels he cannot trust the system and acts in a way that is self-protective rather than letting labor continue without interference, it costs us. When we trust birth but no one else in the system we are working in does, it costs us.

We don't do this work because we are martyrs. We do this work because we are willing to pay the price. We know it makes a difference to this mother, this baby, and this family. We know that our presence will reassure nurses and doctors to allow this mother to labor another hour because she is cared for. We know that the price we pay is a drop in the bucket to what is gained by everyone else by our presence. We do birth doula work because we are called to make a difference in the world.

Our spirit yearning for expression in the world says, "Yes!"

This is your role.

Be of service.

Make a difference.

Hold the spirit alive.

Like a soft spring breeze it whispers, "*Doula this world —it needs you.*"

Another Reason Why Birth Is Sacred

Long ago I learned that rescuing people from their own actions is often a trap, one that ensnares us as well as the person we are trying to help. When it comes to my client's birth it can be really hard as they make decisions that are not going to take them in the direction that was previously desired. As a doula I want to grab them and say, "No! Nooo….No!" The more attached I am to them personally the harder it is…until I shift my thinking. Once I remind myself to respect the transformation and challenges of pregnancy and birth as a sacred path it becomes much easier to support and serve this person.

Several decades ago there was a lot of interest in vision quests* and understanding the deeper spiritual nature of existence. People entered these journeys of challenge and hardship to discover their strengths, weaknesses, inner nature, and relationship to the Divine. For some groups it also involved the risk of death. Joseph Campbell wrote extensively about the "hero's journey" and the meaning and interpretations of this myth in contemporary society. (Today we have Frodo and Harry Potter.)

Early on in my path as a doula, I saw the potential of birth to hold these same meanings for today's women. Women face these same challenges by gestating, giving birth, and nursing – they didn't need a vision quest in the wilderness. While our culture has not adopted the idea of a ritualized journey, the experience of childbirth still holds this potential for women. I suspect it is the same for Trans persons. But that is their story to tell. My labor support has been with cisgendered women so that is the place where I am speaking from.

If we appreciate a woman's birth story as her own personal myth it has the potential to reveal to her deep truth and knowing about herself. It can be a mirror of who she is. Within her birth story is how she deals with challenge, how she deals with authority, how she supports herself, what strengths she brings forth that she didn't know she had. It reveals her relationship to what is unknowable and undefinable in human existence. She must give herself over to a process that may be unknown to her that she is not in control of. How does she respond? What allies does she call upon? When the crisis comes, what does she do? How does she deal with her deep fear as it faces her in the mirror? How does she experience pain, what does she *want* to do about it and what *does* she do about it? How does this mother see the world? How does she see her place in it?

To me, every laboring woman I am with is traversing this terrain. My role is to guide her to finding her own way not to show her which way is right. There is no way I can know her inner experience or how her history has shaped her to act in these moments. I don't need to know – I just need to trust that this journey is unfolding as it should for her. Women have taught me to trust them to find their own truth.

This doesn't mean it's easy. This doesn't mean I don't speak up; it means I trust her to let me know she wants me to. It means I have learned to ask an important question in response to my internal "No! No!": "Is my feeling about *me* or about *her*?" It means I trust that when she whispers, "I think I want an epidural." I whisper back, "Do you want to talk about it some or do you already know that's what you want?" If she nods "yes", I get the nurse. I believe she KNOWS and I do not rob her of that power of choice. To dither about her birth plan is to diminish her as being able to know what is best for her in that moment. My service is to trust her unconditionally as the heroine on her own quest. She will find herself whether she wants to or not.

In my decades of doulaing I have found that many women come back to me and say that their births taught them so much about themselves. They learned who they were. They faced their fears and lived the consequences of their choices. When a woman has support, true support without an agenda, she finds her voice. We amplify it so others can hear it too.

Women change their lives based on their births. They end bad relationships, become fiercer mothers, move across the country, yell at their obstetricians, yell at their midwives, hug and cry with their obstetricians and their midwives, grieve for not knowing. They grieve for the woman they left behind and embrace the woman they now are. *Who am I to know what is best for that woman in the midst of her birth? I know nothing!*

Acknowledging the deep spiritual nature of birth and the risks it contains for crisis and change, keeps me humble. It also frees me. I am a chosen companion for the journey, an ally who will respond as needed. Sometimes offering wisdom but always offering patience and calm. I follow her lead because this is *Her Story*, the myth she is living and creating with each breath. I trust *Her* and I trust my service to her, which is why birth and the path of doulaing when practiced this way is sacred.

> *"It is by going down into the abyss that we recover the treasures of life. Where you stumble, there lies your treasure."*
> -Joseph Campbell

* The term "vision quest" has different historical and cultural meanings in Native American or First People cultures. I'm using a popular culture definition of the term.

If you wish to explore these ideas further:

The Women's Wheel of Life, Elizabeth Davis* and Carol Leonard, Penguin/Arkana, 1996 (*midwife and author of the midwifery textbook, *Heart and Hands)*

The Wholistic Stages of Labor by Whapio Diane Bartlett http://www.thematrona.com/apps/blog/the-holistic-stages-of-labor-by-whapio

The Woman Who Runs With The Wolves: Myths and Stories of the Wild Woman Archetype by Clarissa Pinkola Estes, Ballantine Books (1993)

Joseph Campbell and the Power of Myth DVD Documentary, *PBS, 1988, 2013*

Transformation Through Birth, Claudia Panuthos, Bergin and Garvey, 1984 (still being published!)

Birthing From Within, Pam England, Partera Press, 1998

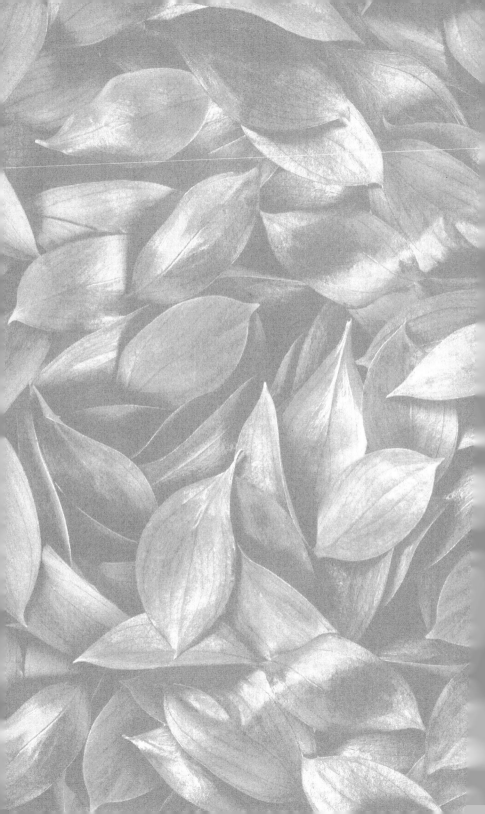

Scope of Practice

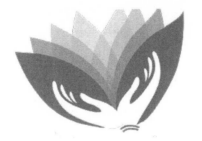

The Essential (Oil) Dilemma

Repeatedly, doulas discuss whether or not it's in their scope of practice to recommend aromatherapy or use essential oils. While that is a part of the discussion, it really isn't the central issue. What we need to recognize is an underlying philosophical difference between doulas. **The core issue is whether it is the doula's role to DO more to moms or just to BE present with her as the labor unfolds.** In the DO camp, people say they want to have more tools in their birth bag. When a few simple sniffs can help with nausea or mood, or even help a person to urinate, that is a good thing. There are so many other interventions happening with the labor, using oils can help to counter them and bring the labor back into balance – or at least make the laboring parent feel better.

The BE group tends to feel that laboring parents have enough people trying to alter the course of their labors. These doulas feel their strength is in the support they bring and the use of comfort measures to alleviate discomfort, not to change what is happening in the labor or what the person is feeling. Being "present with" and supporting the client 100% means not seeing them or their labor as a problem that needs to be fixed. Doulas are usually the only ones who are not trying to will things to be different than what they are. In a postpartum context, these issues are still present. Is it our support that makes a difference or is it the tools we bring to help with post birth discomforts? There is also a baby to consider, whose system may react differently than expected to scents and oils.

The BE-la vs. DO-la* debate isn't new, but it reflects one of the philosophical differences between doulas. I don't think either of these approaches is wrong, but each leads us in a different direction. As a community we haven't formally acknowledged these two approaches. The essential oils issue brings them to the forefront, and offers an effective way to frame this discussion. If you're a DO-la, using essential oils and/or aromatherapy makes sense.

The next issue with essential oils and aromatherapy is more practical. Is there a potential for harm when they are used? The answer is clearly "yes". People can get burned or have unexpected adverse reactions (headache, migraine, nausea, allergic reactions, skin sensitization, photo toxicity, etc.).[1] For example, the desired result of calming a laboring person by using lavender can have the unintended effect of lessening contraction strength and frequency. However, these reactions are not common enough to discourage unwary doulas from buying them. They see themselves as trying to help clients. If you haven't seen an adverse reaction or had one yourself, it's hard to imagine that someone else might.

Essential oils are drugs. They are processed products that are used with the intention of altering what is already occurring. They smell nice, have fun names, and are easily available. You can buy them at parties! But that does not mean they are benign. Rather they are potent substances deserving of respect and care. Many hospitals need to chart their use in labor. For these reasons, using essential oils as an *untrained* doula should be avoided. Some would say that is enough reason for doulas to always leave them alone.

One of the core tenets for almost any doula is that the laboring person should be free to make their own choices, and the doula's role is to fully support them in those choices. Including essential oils and/or aromatherapy as part of one's practice could certainly be one of those choices, if you know what you're doing. It just seems so simple to pair a scent with a relaxation exercise during pregnancy to condition the client to relax when smelling the same scent in early or active labor.

However if you want to use this powerful tool, you need to take full responsibility for it. To me that means informing your client of all the risks of using essential oil therapy as well as the benefits, and having your client acknowledge that in writing.

The risks to the pregnant person if the doula isn't fully informed are great. They are not "safe" for everyone and any web site that makes that claim is wrong. According to one doula, you can be liable for prosecution if there is a negative consequence, depending on how your state's legislation is written. She suggests that the way to protect yourself and your client is to pair with a certified aromatherapist and have them make the recommendations. Then the doula follows through on what the mother wants to do based on the consultation. The risks to our *profession* are even higher. Because doulas are in a tentative position in many communities, and a black mark against one doula who causes harm to a mother can easily tarnish the reputation of doulas in general. I don't want to be alarmist, but our position is precarious in some communities. I often think that newer doulas are not considering how their actions affect everyone else. We live in a global world now. This means you have a responsibility to other doulas and our profession once you begin to use the title of "doula".

These days there's really no excuse for using essential oils without completing a high quality course and engaging in ongoing discussions with others who use oils dermally and as aromatherapy. Birth Arts International offers a self paced course specifically for doulas. As with all things, if the course is being offered by someone who is also selling you a specific brand of products, sales may be their primary motivator. You may not receive objective information from them and they may not have the breadth of experience you'd like in an instructor about their use during pregnancy, labor, and postpartum.

Some doula certifying organizations prohibit the use of essential oils or aromatherapy, taking the stance that they are drugs. Others advocate that interested doulas take formal education or certification so they can be used properly and follow an aromatherapy standard of practice. Yet others have no opinion on the matter. [2] This confuses the average doula who just wants to help their clients. The better we understand what the debate is really about – philosophically, educationally, and professionally, the better we can support each other to find our own right actions.

Note: In the interest of full disclosure, I have used essential oils on several occasions, most notably on my dog when he was dying of untreatable cancer. I would don gloves and a facial mask twice a day and apply the oils in several places on his body. The veterinarian, oil consultant, and I are all convinced that their application made him more comfortable, stimulating his appetite, minimizing his discomfort, and lengthening his life. Second, my body does not respond positively to essential oils. There are very few that do not irritate my skin or cause other unpleasant symptoms, including migraine headaches. However I have close friends and midwives who have been using them in their professional practices with people and animals for a long time. All of them have completed formal educational to gain the knowledge to use them appropriately and safely. Because of these experiences, I have a healthy respect for the power of essential oils.

*Thank you to Gena Kirby and Lesley Everest who introduced me to this phrase.

[1] http://www.agoraindex.org/Frag_Dem/eosafety.html

https://www.naha.org/explore-aromatherapy/safety/

[2] In August 2017 Kim James, owner of www.doulamatch.net counted 67 doula training organizations .

What It Means To Be A Professional Birth Doula

There is a line between doulas who are professionals – where this is the source of their livelihood and the mainstay of their lives next to family and self – and other women who doula occasionally. Not all doulas are professionals nor is it a goal for all doulas. There is a place for all kinds of doulas and we need everyone if we are to reclaim our understanding of birth as important in people's lives. We lost it in the last century and taking a doula training or doulaing friends and family is a way to reclaim that.

Being professional does not diminish the spiritual value we find in our work or the fact that many of us find it to be a calling. We would be diminished in some way if we could not be doulas. We have the joy of being in a life situation that enables us to do work we are passionate about, change the world for another family, and create income at the same time.

In my writings, I frequently use the term "professional doula". It is on a lot of web sites - even in the names of international organizations. But no one has really defined specifically how it applies to our profession. So I analyzed data from my 60 doula interviews, sifted through what I was reading on social media, and read through several books on professionalism. This is what I have come up with to describe the internal identity and behaviors exhibited by doulas who consider themselves professionals. I'd also like to introduce the term "emerging professional", to represent doulas who are growing to meet professional standards. So what does it mean to be a professional doula today?

1. To be a professional means that you have completed education and training to gain the necessary knowledge and skills recognized by others in your profession. Much of doula education is self-study, reading books and completing assignments, combined with taking a workshop and using hands-on skills correctly. Training may involve working with a mentor and on the job training without any supervision. Improvement comes from appraising our experiences and evaluations from clients, nurses, midwives and doctors.

2. To be a professional means you have acquired expert and specialized knowledge. This goes beyond learning a double hip squeeze in a workshop. It means making sense of people's conflicting needs in the birth room; intuiting when to speak and when to keep silent; how to talk to a physician about the patient with a sexual abuse history; how to set up a lap squat with an epidural; and so forth. Competence and confidence grow in interpersonal and labor support arenas. Any additional service you offer to clients means that you have additional study, experience, and possibly mentorship or certification to use it appropriately.

3. To be a professional means that you receive something in return for your services. For many of us that is money or barter goods. However there are doulas who receive stipends that prohibit receiving money for any services performed. They may request a donation be made to an organization instead. If they meet the other requirements for professionalism charging money should not be the sole criteria holding them back.

4. To be a professional means that you market your services and seek out clients that are previously unknown to you. You consider doulaing to be a business.

5. To be a professional means that you hold yourself to the highest standards of conduct for your profession. You seek to empower your clients and not speak for them. You give information but refrain from giving advice. You make positioning and comfort measure recommendations that are in your client's best interests. Your emotional support is unwavering and given freely. Your goal is to enhance communication and connection between her and her careproviders. You seek to meet your client's best interests as she defines them. Several doula organizations have written a code of ethics and/or scope of practice in accordance with their values. They require any doula certifying with them to uphold them. But signing a paper and acting in accordance with those standards are two different things. Even the values represented by various organizations are different. Holding yourself to the highest standards is shown by how *you behave*.

6. To be a professional means that you put your client first. When you make a commitment to be there, you're there. If you become ill or have a family emergency there is another professional who can seamlessly take over for you. You keep your client's information and history confidential. Confidentiality means not posting anything specific or timely on any social media. Your responsibility to their needs takes priority over your own.

7. To be a professional means that you cultivate positive relationships with other perinatal professionals whenever possible. You respect their point of view even when it differs from yours. You seek to increase your communication skills and to understand different cultural perspectives. You keep your experiences with them confidential and private. You learn from past mistakes.

8. To be a professional means that you have experience with a wide variety of births and feel confident in your ability to handle almost anything that comes along. Other professional doulas respect you and make referrals. Note that I did not include a number of births. Because of life and career experiences, some doulas will arrive at this place sooner than others.

9. To be a professional means that you seek out and commit to doula certification that promotes maximum empowerment of the client using non-clinical skills, and values and promotes client-medical careprovider communication. This role requires additional education before offering additional non-clinical skills. Certification means that you are held to standards that people outside your profession can read and understand. Not being certified means there are no set expectations for that doula's behavior. Some doula training organizations have very loose certification standards with no specific behaviors listed, just general attitudes. Certification with behavioral standards that can evaluate whether the doula acted according to those standards is important for furthering the professionalism of birth doula work outside our own individual spheres. It means that a doula is accountable to someone outside of herself and her individual client. (In other words, certification *in the context of professionalism* is not about you, but about how it affects other people's perceptions of you AND our profession as a whole.) Having said this, not all doulas have certification like this available to them.

10. To be a professional means that you seek to improve your profession by serving in organizations, representing your profession at social events, and assisting novice doulas to improve their services. You balance your own desires and needs with the actions

that further the doula profession – such as certification. You know that when you get better – increase your skills, knowledge and integrity – you improve the work environment for *all* labor doulas.

11. To be a professional means that you have personal integrity. Integrity means that your values, what you say, and how you behave are congruent with one another. Sullivan has written:

"Integrity is never a given, but always a quest that must be renewed and reshaped over time. It demands considerable individual self-awareness and self-command…Integrity of vocation demands the balanced combination of individual autonomy with integration to its shared purposes. Individual talents need to blend with the best common standards of performance, while the individual must exercise personal judgment as to the proper application of these communal standards in a responsible way." [p. 220]

"Integrity can only be achieved under conditions of competing imperatives. Unless you are torn between your lawyerly duties as a zealous advocate for your client and your communal responsibilities as an officer of the court, you cannot accomplish integrity. Unless you are confronted with the tensions inherent in the practice of any profession, the conditions for integrity are not present: "Integrity is not a given…."

In a doula context, this means that when you are in the labor room trying to figure out what the right thing is to do and struggling with it, you are having a crisis of integrity. "Do I say something to the medical careprovider (MCP) or do I keep my mouth shut? Have the parents said anything on their own behalf? Do I just let this happen and help them afterwards?" What value takes precedent: empowerment of the client or allowing an intervention to occur that may affect the course of the labor? How will each potential action change my relationship with the MCP? Situations like these are true tests of integrity that require us to rank our values of what is most important.

Sullivan, William M. (2nd ed. 2005). *Work and Integrity: The Crisis and Promise of Professionalism in America*. Jossey Bass.

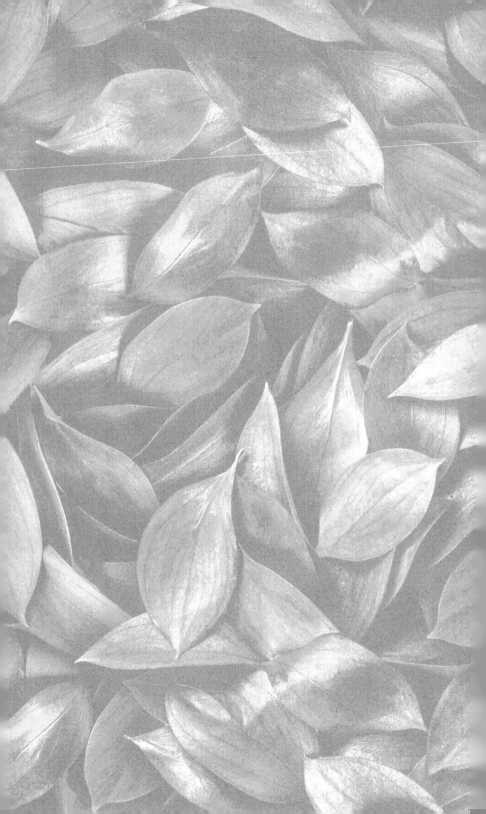

Clients

Why Mothers Choose
A Particular Doula

Let's say you are a woman and have a problem where you need some advice. Explaining the situation will require some self-disclosure and revealing personal information. You are in a meeting for the day with women you have never met before. The advice you need can't wait so you'll need to choose to reveal your problem to one of the women present. As the day goes on you have the opportunity to observe and interact with everyone. When you make your choice, what are you likely to base it on? Is it the intellectual qualities or resume of the person? Or the woman you feel comfortable enough to disclose your feelings and your dilemma? If you're like most women, it will be the person you feel safest with.

The same thing is true about how a mother chooses her doula. It is based on her gut feeling - who she can be naked with - because she will be. Who she senses can accept her fears and her lifestyle – because that is our role. All of these attributes are due to who *the mom is*: what she intuits as right for her, which we as doulas cannot influence at all. **A woman's gut feeling about which doula is right for her has more to do with who that woman is than who we are.**

That mom may need a mother, a sister, or a new friend who knows a lot about birth. She may need someone she can say "no" to safely. But whatever it is she needs, choosing a doula is an emotional decision not an intellectual one. Mothers say, "It just felt right." "I felt safe with her." "I just knew she was the one." "I was leaning towards another doula but wasn't sure. Then I met our doula and something clicked."

"Even though she didn't look as good as the others on paper, we just connected and that was it."

Effective doulas are nurturers and good listeners. In an initial interaction, these are the qualities that attract someone to you. After that, it is all about anticipating and meeting the mother's needs – and we don't yet know what they are. She may not even be able to put them into words, but that doesn't mean that her brain isn't communicating them on some level. Often the brain sends emotional information to the nerve endings in the digestive system.[1] Her gut feeling about who is right for her is just that.

I often find myself reassuring new doulas about getting clients. It isn't about the best web site or the number of workshops you've attended. It doesn't matter whether you have given birth yourself. Parents choose doulas based on a number of criteria. Yes, cost and experience do count. Some parents enjoy cool websites with professional photos. But mothers are often looking for someone they can have an intimate relationship with.

Which is why I think competition between doulas is unnecessary. It is more important to be yourself and work on developing your interpersonal skills and a nonjudgmental attitude. When we compete with other doulas in our community we may diminish the opportunities for all of us to get clients. When we band together to promote doula support and have inclusive "Meet The Doula" events, we send a positive cooperative message to other birth professionals and prospective clients.

[1] http://www.scientificamerican.com/article.cfm?id=gut-second-brain

Why Not To Share
Your Birth Story

A major part of our effectiveness as doulas is being authentically ourselves without revealing a lot of information about our lives. We are most effective doulaing our clients when we can be whoever she needs us to be. The less they know about us, the easier that is. We are free to shape ourselves around our client and her family. Good doulaing has much more to do with who we are being in the present moment with our clients than our lifestyle choices or personal history.

The easiest way to start is to set good professional boundaries and not include personal details that aren't important to your doula-client relationship. Such as not having meetings at your home – have them either at the client's home or a neutral place. What your partner does or your children's interests or even your housekeeping standards are all unrelated to your ability to be a good doula. Yet, your pregnant client will take that information into account in evaluating you and your abilities to assist their family. So my recommendation is to take it out of the equation.

Conducting my thesis and doctoral research reinforced for me that it is not a good idea to share your own pregnancy and birth stories with your clients. None of my own clients has any idea what my births were like or the decisions I made. It is completely irrelevant and gets in the way of her allowing me in. Pregnant clients can be notoriously self-judgmental. They may compare themselves to others to find out whether their own decisions are "better" or "worse". Our clients do this – sometimes when we tell them the story or later during the labor as they make their own choices. As doulas, our clients consider us experts – thus our choices carry more weight with them. Many doulas have had a laboring person turn to them and sob, "What will you think of me if I do this?" So I keep silent about my own journey.

This can be a dilemma for doulas who are also childbirth educators (CBE). Sharing about births in an education situation has a different purpose – "Learn from what I know". Childbirth educators are also freer to advocate for certain choices. When the CBE is hired as a doula, she needs to be prepared to deal with this issue directly and be more aware of the potential impact on the mother during labor. I heard this from every mother who hired her childbirth educator as a doula in my study: "I wondered what she was thinking of me".

As a doula, when a mother asks me, *"What were your births like?"* I turn it around. For doulas who have not given birth, *"What would you do?"* is the same question. *"Tell me more about why you would like to know."* It could be they are interested in getting to know me better; then it is easy to redirect to another topic to build intimacy. It could be they are trying to figure out a dilemma. In that instance, I can offer more information or some more emotional support. In either case, asking about my births is often metaphorical; it is a question that indicates my client is seeking care. Their underlying needs will be better met in other ways than discussing my births. In our own heads we need to understand that the question about our births may not be about our births at all. It is an indicator that there is a need and my client isn't sure how to express it. Our job is to figure out what it is and how to meet it.

I'm not advocating you never say anything – there are very few things that are absolutes in the doula guidebook! Sometimes it is very simple. "Did you have a long labor like I did?" is just that – they want to know if I have faced the same challenge. "No, but I have attended a lot of people who did and helped them through it." Short answer plus emotional support – we aren't dwelling on our stories, but meeting the underlying need as we perceive it. However, we need to know that laboring person pretty well and sometimes we're still wrong. "Tell me more about why you'd like to know" can give us so much rich information about our clients! It invites them to reflect on themselves and learn something – sometimes something significant. Rather than assuming we already know, their answer tells us so much more about how we can best meet their needs.

The really important thing is to be conscious about what you share about yourself and to make sure that information is in your and your client's best interests. You need to know them pretty well in order to choose what to say. Remember this is a professional relationship, not a friendship. You want to build intimacy and safety, but they are engaging you for a service. Based on my research and years of experience, pregnant people and their families want be accepted exactly as they are – that is part of your support role. Since people automatically compare themselves to others, you want to make sure that the information you share will soften those comparisons.

Now I know there are doulas who share their personal stories on their web sites – they feel it is honest and a significant part of the way they doula. However, it is likely that they attract clients who agree with their choices or feel attracted to the emotions expressed in their story. This is not bad, only limiting. People probably self select whether to email or call based on reading the story. It really depends on the doula, the kind of clients they want to attract, and the kind of practice they have. The key message I am making is to be conscious about your choices in what you share, to realize it has hidden impacts, and that mother's questions are often not what they seem to be on the surface.

Showing Up

One of the doula research interviews that influenced me profoundly happened at a 2004 conference. That morning a birth colleague, Sophie*, came striding in to my hotel room with coffee and her breakfast on a plate. We'd met in 1988 at a retreat for birth professionals.

"I didn't think you'd mind if I ate while we talked," she said as her plate clunked down on the glass table. When I transcribed the interview later, I could hear her chewing and cutting her lox and bagel with a knife and fork on the recording. It was so like Sophie to assume my loving acceptance of her quirks, just like she would expect to accept mine.

I turned on the recorder. With her first story, Sophie said, "Amy, the most important thing you do isn't a double hip squeeze. It's not whether she gets drugs. It's showing up. Showing up is 50% of what we do as doulas."

As the interview progressed, she told more stories and reflected on what she'd learned. Sophie said, "I change that! Showing up is 75 % of what we do as doulas!"

By the end of the two hour interview, she changed her mind again.

"It's 99% of what we do as doulas! The rest is just fluff. Showing up for her, that is what counts."

Showing up is an approach of non-judgment and a series of continuing actions over time that support the mother wholeheartedly even when others are unable to accept or support the mother's needs (Gilliland, 2004).

In my research, doulas who had been to a hundred or more births usually told stories about this deep level of acceptance, or what Sophie called "showing up", as being the most important and most significant service that the doula can offer. Many proficient and expert doulas mentioned the need to accept mothers whatever they are feeling or doing, and to believe them when they say they want something, even if it is different from their stated wishes prior to labor. Here's the excerpt from my original interview with Sophie:

"In my life there is always compromise, always negotiation, always other people in mind. I have to take everybody else into consideration. So I think when someone shows up for me one hundred percent, supports me one hundred percent, hears everything I have to say and amplifies it, that's what I mean by *showing up*. That to me is the greatest gift. That's it. I think that's 99%. I'm going up to ninety-nine. [laughs heartily] I think that's huge. I really do. Because I think very few women get to have that."

Women have to compromise for everyone in their life. They have to compromise for their partners, for their kids, for their pets, for their parents, bosses, and on and on. **Women shouldn't have to compromise for their doula at their own birth**! Instead our role is to be present and mindful in the moment, and do that for hours and hours, answering her needs so she is free to labor. What she says she wants, even if it's surprising, isn't there to be challenged. Explored and confirmed, yes, not challenged. Additionally, when women feel that whatever they do or say or how they behave will be acceptable to their doula, they will feel free to enter fully into their experience of birthing their baby.

What does that look like? Let's say I'm at a birth, with a mom who had previously been adamant about not using pain medication. She looks at me and for whatever reason, says, "I think I want an epidural." The doula's "showing up" thought process prompts me to consider the mom and ask, "What can I do to best support her in this moment?" The attitude of the doula has to be one of caring detachment. If we get caught up in our clients doing things a certain way or having certain things happen, the experience becomes about us and not about them. Effective doulas need to find a way to be caring and loving of the woman and her intimate family, without being attached to what she does, how she makes decisions, or what choices she makes. It's essential for our own mental health, but also for our effectiveness as labor support.

What do I say to that mom? "Would you like to talk about it more or try something else first, or do you want me to get the nurse?" If she says to get the nurse, then that's it. I'm there to support the woman in labor, not her birth plan.

But the reality for us is that we WANT things for our clients, we WANT them to have great births, we DO get attached. What helps me is understanding that the birth is her journey; she is the leader, she tells me the route. If I think she's making a "wrong" turn, that is me comparing her journey with some idealized one I have in my head. I know birth influences the course of women's lives forevermore. So who am I to judge what's best? I don't know her path. When I can say that inside of me and really own it, I am much freer to support a wide variety of women making a wide variety of choices, and to truly *show up* for them.

*her name has been changed

Gilliland, A.L. (2004) Effective labor support by doulas. In *Human development and family studies*, Vol. Master's Thesis. University of Wisconsin-Madison, Madison, pp. 276.

The Art Of Labor Sitting

Labor sitting is the process of being present with a person while they are laboring; they don't require your direct attention, but do need you to be attentive. In other words, labor is going well but there really is nothing for the doula to do but step to the outer circle and wait. Common situations for labor sitting are early labor, the first few hours of an induction, when person is resting with an epidural, or taking turns with another member of the birth team.

Good labor sitting means that the doula seems occupied but interruptable. The person in labor does not feel pressured by your presence to be further along in labor or to be doing anything different than what they are doing. At the same time your presence is felt, knowing you are available if needed. Often, labor sitting takes place in the same room. Effective labor sitting is an active, not passive process. It may seem we are sitting on the couch working on a little project. But a good doula is much more aware of what is going on than it seems!

So how do you strike this balance? Over the years, through trial and error – doing it wrong and by accident doing it right and then repeating it – I have found my way to effective labor sitting. I do needlepoint. If I were reading a book or looking at the screen on my phone, I would seem occupied by what I was doing. My attention would be focused on the book or my phone. Someone might feel they were interrupting me if they spoke to me. If I am just sitting there, people might feel bad because I'm just sitting in the chair not doing anything. They might feel pressured because my skills weren't being used yet. If I am sitting on the couch doing needlepoint*, my mind is in the room with them, yet I am happily occupied.

One time a father called me saying he and his female partner were getting ready to go to the hospital. They weren't packed yet so he was rushing around the house. Her contractions were 4-5 minutes apart with no bloody show. She was relaxing in the bathtub and coping well. Through our conversation I got the idea that Dad was anxious. I surmised he wanted to go to the hospital because it would relieve his anxiety. As we've all learned from TV when you go to the hospital the baby comes out. While this is an irrational belief, it is the way our culture has trained us.

I offered to come over and help. When I arrived, the pregnant partner had just gotten out of the tub and gave me a big smile. My doula assessment of the labor was that it was not time to go to the hospital. I asked her preference and she said she wasn't ready to go (she is the decider, not me). We talked a bit and I went to sit on the couch and got out my needlepoint. I didn't say anything but after a while Dad seemed to calm down. We chatted and his furious pace of grabbing household items and putting them in a pile slowed down. He began to pay more attention to his partner. The message he got from my behavior was: "Amy's calm so there must not be any rush." When she had a contraction I would stop and breathe with her, looking at her from across the room. This visual regard is also a part of effective labor support – if she were to look at me she would see that I was watchful and available. In due time we went to the hospital; they were both calm and made the decision they were ready.

Another time labor sitting skills come in handy is at the beginning of an induction. There are many anxieties to soothe and many decisions that are made in those first few hours that have repercussions later. If I am present I am able to remind them of their choices, make sure their questions are answered, and calm them down. I create an atmosphere in the room to make it their space. I can increase the level of connection between my client and the nurse, resident physician, and attending physician. If I am not there, those things often do not happen. This is another time to discuss methods of induction and parent's concerns. It is often easier to advocate for using the shower or tub, or having a slower, gradual Pitocin drip before any interventions are administered. Parents may be able to get approval for a plan to go home under certain conditions. What I have found most often is that a pregnant person may bring up these things and then the medical care providers (MCP) explain why they won't do it that way. But in the long run, my client has explored their options to the extent they wanted to. Plus, the MCP and my client have talked and understand each other's concerns and preferences. The nurse has heard the client and can suggest other suitable labor support or intervention suggestions.

Of course discussing options is about fifteen minutes out of three hours of labor sitting. Even if none of these discussions happen, your client may have other fears on their minds and other choices to be made. I have never found **NOT** being there at the beginning of an induction to gain my clients or me anything. Sometimes with a Pitocin induction, parents want me to leave for a while. That's fine and we agree to check in verbally – not with a text – every hour or two. If they want privacy with a misoprostol induction, I stay immediately outside the room or return every 15-20 minutes. Those intense contractions may start without warning and the partner or nurse may not be able to contact me.

Labor sitting is a creative art. It requires understanding the people involved; being able to forecast possible futures, and an empathetic, compassionate presence. This is not a passive process – you are *not* waiting for something to happen and then responding to it. Instead, you are influencing the present moment. You are there, caring, mindful, and available. People take their cues from your behavior and from your presence. Because of active compassionate labor sitting, labor often unfolds differently.

Some doulas embroider or crochet something for the baby or make a lace cap out of a handkerchief. If you're a knitter, you may wish to use needles that don't click.

Why You Should Keep
Your Hands To Yourself

nswer: "Vaginal exams." Jeopardy question: "What is one thing
a doula does not do?" Most of us hear these reasons in our doula
trainings: doulas are not experienced at it; it introduces germs; it is a
medical diagnosis (liability); or that it "muddies the waters" between
the doula's role and that of other medical professionals. There are doulas and other birth professionals who feel that doing vaginal exams at
home in early labor is an advantage. When I first started as a labor assis-
tant in the mid-1980's it was assumed that I would someday provide
vaginal exams and other clinical skills. We thought being able to offer
more medical information to the pregnant person would be empowering. After years of personal experience and research, I now theorize it is
more empowering for our clients and more powerful for the doulas to
avoid doing vaginal exams. Here's why:

1. Everyone else wants to put their fingers in our client's vagina!
    Triage nurses, doctors, residents, midwives, midwifery students,
    nursing students, you name it. Even though a cervical check may
    seem useful when trying to gauge when to go from home to the
    hospital, doing vaginal exams doesn't help me be a better doula. I
    just become another person who is entering the private spaces of
    a pregnant person's body.

2. Doing so changes the balance of power in the client doula rela-
    tionship away from an act of service. As a doula my role is to
    empower and support this person one hundred percent. If they

want something I help them to get it; if they don't want something I help them to say "no". My role is to help my clients believe in themselves. As a professional doula, I have no agenda other than to support them and their loved ones. As people we are equals and I am there to serve them as they labor and birth their child.

Once I put my hand inside of their body we are no longer equals – they don't put their hand in my vagina. The social roles between us have shifted. In their mind *who I am* symbolically has changed. I used to be there to serve them and now I have touched them intimately and evaluated their body! This shifts the power balance between us so that I have more power than they do – I have personal private knowledge of their body they do not have of mine (and very likely will never have). Our support relationship is no longer the same.

3.   With that one act, the doula role shifts from support to evaluation. I am judging their body. I am giving them information about themselves that we don't believe they have any other way. I am subtly communicating that I don't trust them to know where they are in labor. Their intuitive knowledge of their own body and labor isn't good enough – we need to check the cervix just to be sure.

4.   The doula misses the opportunity to empower the mother. When you aren't doing the evaluating, you need to rely on the mother's internal messages. She lives in her own body, for goodness' sake, which is something most people tend to forget. You can call it intuition or receptivity to subtle nerve signals perceived by the brain. The mother has access to what is going on in her body and as a doula I can assist her to listen to these messages. If we can help her to identify what she is experiencing and feeling, she can

discern for herself what she wants to do. When we model early on: "It's your body, what do you feel? What do you want to do?", it starts a pattern that can carry on throughout her labor.

5.   Not relying on vaginal exams means that the doula hones other observational skills. Patterns of breathing, skin color changes, cartilage and bone changes, even the usual bloody show and contraction patterns can all tell us where the mother is in labor. Combined with her own internal messages we can present her with information so she can decide. We can also observe signs of progressing labor, dehydration, or other concerns which might lead us to think that going to the hospital or birth center is a good idea.

As doulas, our very presence is an effort to put the mother at the center of her own birth experience. Our role of unconditional non-invasive support is unique. No one else can offer what the doula does. Rather than being a limitation, avoiding vaginal exams empowers both the mother and the doula. Why endanger that when the price can be so high?

*Having said that, there are some clients that really want at home labor support that includes vaginal exams. That is why there are monitrices who possess both clinical skills and labor support skills and are covered by midwifery or nursing standards of care. There are also midwives who will teach the mother's intimate life partner to get to know her cervix during pregnancy so they can feel for labor changes. But the expectations that are brought to the midwifery relationship and nursing relationship are different than with professional doula support.

Being Who She Needs You To Be – When It's Easy

O ne of the significant concepts that arose out of my doula research was the enduring theme of shifting how you doula-ed in order to meet the needs of different people. On the surface, this seems like a deceptively simple concept: different mothers have different needs. Some women need a sister, some a mother, some a grandmother, some a new birth knowledgeable friend. As I've said before, women hire you based on what they need - which is an intuitive process. She already senses you have the potential to fulfill her needs. What comes next is a *process* of adapting one's skills and communications to best meet those needs. You can think of "being whoever she needs me to be" as a description of *HOW you doula* a mother. Maybe you can relate to these two doulas' words:

Doula A: *"I will match the energy in the room. I will match their moods. I will take on the music that they're listening to. I will join in the conversations that they're discussing. I will ask more about their life because I want to know more about them, I may pray with them. But I don't think I actually lose my inner self. My inner self actually connects with their inner selves."*

Doula B: *"It's taking your cues from them, picking up on the energy and just relating to them in whatever capacity they need. Sometimes I'm an information giver and I don't do anything hands-on because they want that between them. Sometimes the dad doesn't want to do anything hands-on, and I'm totally hands-on. And sometimes they don't want the information because they have all the information that they believe they need in their heads. So it really depends totally on the couple."*

When I was analyzing my first few doula interviews, this concept arose spontaneously. After that, I heard almost every experienced doula describe it. Later on, I selected passages from over 40 interviews and analyzed them, grouping similar ideas together. From that I've been able to outline this process and come to understand that sometimes 'being whoever she needs you to be' is very satisfying, and other times it can hurt you down to your core. First I want to focus on the process and when it is easy to be the doula she needs.

Emotional support, physical support, informational support and empowerment – these are the four cornerstones of how doulas support mothers. The doula is sensing what the mother and her partner need and being as effective as possible in providing good care. But it is the mother who is shaping the doula, who is bringing out of the doula what is inside to meet her needs. Most of the time we enter a labor room curious about how the labor will unfold and not knowing what will be demanded of us. We just roll with whatever comes our way. Because we are adapting our skills to meet their needs, parents get to determine what roles we play in their lives. We extend ourselves in a position of service for them – and they get to choose how they wish us to serve.

My research showed several fairly common roles or needs expressed by different mothers or their doulas. Doulas did not struggle at all with these functions. Here, different doulas describe roles that are common and easy to adapt to. Sometimes mothers want the doula to be the person who provides:

Informational Support and Empowerment: *"This mom said, "I don't want any of this hippie-dippy stuff. I need answers. I need someone who will help me ask the right questions and gather information."*

Forceful Guidance: *"I think she needed to have a strong person who wouldn't back down when she resisted and said, "Oh, but I'm so comfortable here." She needed someone who would insist that she move around and do things to make the labor more effective."*

Sometimes I'll hear the partner in the other room say, "[The doula] said you have to get out of bed and take a shower. Because she said you're going to feel much better. So let's go." And then two seconds later they're in the shower and Mom's going, "Oh, my God, I can't believe I didn't want to, this is so much better."

Physical Strength: *"Right now I probably couldn't pick up that television, but at a birth I could hold you up as long as you needed me to. It's amazing! I am an amazingly strong person at a birth. I am that kind of a doula. I will sit up in a bed behind her and push with her. I will catch her puke. I mean, I know doulas who won't catch puke. I'll catch her puke. I'll do anything. I will do anything."*

Comforting Presence: *"As soon as I walked in the door, her husband left, went home, 'the construction guys were coming'. It was me and the woman, and I sat there and I held her hand. She was sitting in the rocking chair, and I knelt in front of her, and basically what I did was, I staved off the people who were coming by every 20 minutes or so asking if she wanted medication, which she never did even though they gave her the pitch. She never took an epidural or any other medication. Put a sign on the door and said, "Leave us alone." And then literally all I did was hold that woman's hand. She would open her eyes and look at me. And she would close her eyes back, and I sat there and held her hand. And she told me afterward* *she could not have done it without me. Amy, all I did was hold her hand. I did <u>nothing</u>. I didn't do a comfort measure. I did* nothing.*"*

<u>Acceptance and Humor:</u> *"They were an Orthodox Jewish couple. So her husband could not be there for the actual birth. But he sat behind a curtain and prayed. At one point I said, like from the Wizard of Oz, "Pay no attention to that man behind the curtain!" And oh, I'd never say that to anyone else!"*

<u>To Let Her Lead:</u> *"I'm thinking we're in for a long night because she is so high need so early. She doesn't sound like she's having coping related responses to what's going on at 1-2 centimeters. But she was not willing to relax, and she's not going to sleep anyway no matter what I try to do positioning wise or massaging or whatever. She's not gonna sleep so we might as well work. And that's where she was at. She did not want to relax enough to try and fall asleep, which I felt would benefit her labor - if she would relax and let go."*

Many of these roles or needs could not have been predicted. While we might know that we are expected to help with position changes, what we don't know is whether she will be resistant or not to our suggestions. We don't know if simply sitting with her will be all she needs or we'll be exhausted from walking, stroking, massaging and holding her up. While we always strive to follow the mother's lead, there are times when sleep might be better than activity. But we have to figure out what is more important – her being in charge or the textbook idea to rest. How we give encouragement also shifts. When a woman needs mothering or grandmothering, our responses are different than when she is acting logical and practical. People are very different from one another. A good doula responds by "becoming whoever she needs you to be".

Being Who She Needs You To Be – When It's Difficult

...ᕙᕙᕙᕙᕙᕙᕙᕙᕙᕙᕙᕙᕙᕙᕙᕙᕙᕙᕙᕙᕙᕙᕙᕙᕙᕙᕙᕙᕙᕙᕙᕙᕙᕙ...

Most of us are concerned about mothers not being able to use the bathtub, take a fetal monitor break, delay cord clamping, or labor for a VBAC. Beneath all of this is the fundamental truth of doula work: we enter a woman's life being a guide as she finds her way through one of her life's most challenging journeys. For our clients, birth can be physically, psychologically, mentally, and spiritually challenging. It may be full of anxiety and conflicting messages from family members and medical caregivers. As doulas, we have agreed to provide support that is unencumbered by past history or future expectations. We desire little but that she be true to herself – as she defines it. That is what doula work is all about.

Some clients keep us at a distance. Others bring us into their drama and thrust us into playing a part we would not have chosen for ourselves. We become what they need to get through labor. This can sometimes be awkward, unexpected, and challenging. Have you ever been to a birth and wondered, *"What is going on here? What does she expect me to do? I'm not sure how to handle this or what to say."* Odds are you are being thrust into a role where 'being who she needs you to be' is uncomfortable. Sometimes it is painful the way some situations turn out – especially when the doula hasn't done anything wrong. This can happen to any doula no matter what their experience level, if they have prenatal visits or meet their clients in labor. It is the laboring mother who chooses the depth of the contact and meaning of her doula in her life.

I came to these conclusions after analyzing dozens of formal research interviews and then checking out my ideas informally with other doulas. Here doulas describe some situations where meeting the mother's needs was difficult.

<u>Family Member:</u> *"She told me at the beginning that I reminded her of the sister that she never had. Meanwhile she does have a sister so I don't know what it was. I think she just took me on as the role of a family member. She saw me more of a friend than as a doula. I was invited to her birthday party and she'd just stop by my house. 'I was just seeing if you were home', kind of thing."*

This doula was cast in the role of family member during her client's pregnancy. This can be an awkward situation and uncomfortable role. The doula needed to figure out where the boundaries needed to be but also needed to understand whether her client was lonely and what was going on. It is really hard to set a boundary after its already been breached especially if the mother is emotionally fragile or needy. Figuring out the appropriate response requires good observation on the doula's part plus sophisticated communication skills. Another possibility is that the doula likes the mother too and wants to become friends. But if they became friends could she be a good doula? With friends one is emotionally involved and there are future expectations.

<u>Hostess Mom's Guest:</u> *"My client says, "Did you all have a good time at my birth?" And I said, "A good time at your birth? What would it be to have a good time at your birth?" She says, "Well, did you all eat anything? Did you have fun?" Then I kind of thought, 'Hmm, did she want to hostess? Did she want us to have a party and have a good time?' So I said, "When you were laboring in that other room, we were in here having a slumber party. It was like a group of girls having this wonderful slumber party." And the delight came out. "Oh! I'm so glad, I so wanted you to have fun at my birth!"*

Although the Hostess mom is rare, I have run into her a few times. She may have difficulty getting into her labor. She wants to make sure the people she cares about are settled and enjoying themselves. Do they have food? Something to do? Will they nap? She may have packed food for the hospital to please everyone else. Instead of focusing inward, she becomes overly concerned with what's going on in her environment. This mom requires patience, reassurance about her loved ones and doula's state of being, and refocusing on laboring. She may be overly quiet because she doesn't want to disturb someone else (part of her "be a good girl" upbringing).

Permission Giver: *"There are a lot of people who kind of just need someone to tell them that getting some kind of help or accepting some intervention or pain medication is not a sign of weakness. For someone to say, "You know what? A really strong person does whatever needs to be done to get the job done. And I understand how you didn't want an epidural, but I'm wondering if you are at your limit and feel bad saying so."*

Sometimes a mother refuses pain medication when she is obviously suffering because she is holding on to some ideal. She does not give herself permission to shift from the vision she set for herself of how she was going to respond in labor. Often we reassure, validate feelings, and reframe. We subtly try to help the mother to find her own truth and make her own choice. But sometimes what she really wants is her doula telling her it's okay *with us.* This can be uncomfortable for the doula because we don't want that kind of power. Remember it is *the mother who looks to the doula for permission* – not the doula who feels she is in the position of giving it. It has been assigned to us – we did not seek it out.

Scapegoat: *"Second stage was very confusing. At one point, she had said something like my mom should leave. I looked at her and said, "Do you want your mom to go now or do you want her to stay?" And she said,*

"Well I think she ought to go." I said, "We can have the nurse say something." I looked at the dad and said, "You heard her. Do you want to talk with the nurse?" So the nurse comes over and they tell her quietly. I didn't say anything. The nurse said to the grandmother, "Why don't we all kind of chill out and you go get some drinks or something to eat." So she missed the birth. Then at the postpartum visit, the mom says, "I never said I wanted my mother to leave. I wished you hadn't told the nurse to tell her to go." There was another doula there too and she was shocked. After trying to explain what happened from my perspective, I realized I should just shut up and apologize. Basically in order for her and her husband and the mother to all come out okay with one another they had to blame it on me."

Unfortunately I have heard more than one version of this story. It is much easier to blame the doula than it is to take personal responsibility. We all know people who don't take responsibility for their own behavior. People don't stop being who they are just because they are in labor. As doulas we have very little power. We are also leaving that family's life. So scapegoating the doula can be a mechanism for making the family members feel safe with one another again. Other scapegoating examples: The partner remains uninvolved with labor support no matter what strategies the doula uses to involve them. The partner showed no initiative and resisted the doula's overtures. Then the doula gets blamed for the partner not behaving as desired. In another case, an intervention does not turn out favorably. The doula may hear: "Why didn't you make sure I knew that could happen?" or "You should have told me not to do it – that's why I hired you."

Someone she can say "no" to: *No matter what you suggest, she says "no". As in, "No, I don't want to ask any more questions. No, I don't want to move. No, I don't want to drink anything. No, I don't like the way you're touching me."* As doulas we sometimes feel frustrated because of the mother's contrariness and our inability to please someone. Sometimes, this mom is testing your support or begging for acceptance. She wants to know that no matter how obstinate or uncooperative she is, you will be there for her. Perhaps she has been let down in the past and really needs the experience of unconditional support.

Another possibility is this mom feels she has little power in her everyday life. She may have to compromise for everyone else and do what others want. However, in labor this mom has permission to say "no". But she may only be able to do that to someone who has no authority and where there will be no consequences afterwards. In effect, she engaged your services in order to be able to use you to meet her psychological needs. Which in this case is to have some power over somebody else – even if her choices are not leading her to the kind of birth experience she previously said she wanted.

People are complicated psychological creatures. When we enter into this path of service for them, we are entering into a relationship where the mother has control. This is necessary in order for us to be effective as doulas and to individualize the care people need. But it doesn't always feel good to be in the roles people cast us. Sometimes it feels that we've been misunderstood or betrayed in some way. We may end up not liking this birth very much.

This is usually a shock for newer doulas. Often they haven't heard these kinds of stories or never really believed them. A new doula may think, "If I only doulaed correctly, then I would not feel inadequate or be blamed." They are not likely to say anything to their doula friends because they think there is something wrong with *them* when that isn't true. In this way our discussion about doula work needs to shift. This is caregiving work that can involve a deep intimacy with our clients and their psychological needs. We become mirrors for their deepest selves. But when they don't like what they see, they may tell us we're the ones who are wrong. We need to have compassion for the difficult situations we find ourselves in. We also need to open up and discuss these situations safely with our colleagues if we are to continue to provide this valuable and important service.

The Time To Ask About Past Abuse Or Assault Is Never

O ne of the most upsetting questions I have read on a doula's personal history form is some version of this: "Have you ever experienced sexual abuse or assault, either as a child or as an adult?" While
I realize the doula is trying to be helpful, the attempt is misguided
at best, and can actually create problems and stresses for the client
that negatively affect the doula-client relationship. What the doula
really wants to know is whether there are ways to help the client more
effectively, even if what the client wants may seem odd or unusual.
There are better ways to obtain that information that don't create more
problems.

Asking the question automatically puts your client in a bind. They
have to choose whether to be honest with you before they are ready to
do so, or whether to lie. The issue with most survivors of abuse or assault
is that the perpetrator took away their power of choice. Their body
was not their own, it was the property of the perpetrator. The victim's
only choice was to submit or possibly face worse harm if they resisted.
Part of offering healing is for us to allow the client to self-disclose if it
is desired, and when they initiate it. When we ask the question, it is
to meet our own needs even though it is in the guise of good intentions. If we ask, this could stimulate their PTSD symptoms because
we're invading our client's day with memories they likely work hard to
avoid. If our client does not wish to discuss these acts or even for us to
know, their only other option is to lie. This dilemma is distressing for
our client, which is not the doula's intention. So don't ask.

The truth is, what you really want to know is how you can help them best through their birth or postpartum journey. There are ways to get at that information without knowing exactly why. In fact, knowing details about the story is not necessary to offering effective support. Below are two possible approaches to get at what you really want to know. Make sure you have established a rapport with your client first. What approach is better to use will depend on the client, the doula, and the situation. The most important guideline is that we want our client to feel empowered and supported throughout the whole conversation with us. Some people don't want to us to know about their difficult past; so any remark that would allude to it is not helpful. Others feel that labeling their past experience as traumatic and having their doula validate that is empowering. So which approach is better varies a great deal. When in doubt, use a gentle and general approach and let the client lead the conversation.

The first conversation starter is gentle and more general. It is a simpler approach that downplays where the preference may have come from.

"Everybody has different preferences for how they like to interact with people. It helps me if I know yours. I don't need to know why and they won't seem strange to me – I'm used to working with all kinds of people. [Pause] Some people want to be asked before they are touched. Others want medical people to use their name and not be called "Mom" or "Sweetie". Sometimes people have a strong need for privacy – they don't want strangers walking in the labor room. We can put a sign up telling them to knock and introduce themselves when they first come in so you're not surprised by who is there. What is important to you?"

The second approach is more direct and specifically mentions the type of experiences we are alluding to:

"Sometimes people have had life experiences that left them trauma-tized and that they had to recover from. Sometimes that involves being in a car accident or natural disaster, or assault or abuse. There may be things that other people do or say that lead you to being instantly scared or startled or remind you of bad memories. I just want you to know that I can help you best when I can help myself and others to avoiding saying or doing those things, and also what to do if they happen."

You can also offer examples:

- *Sometimes a person is easily startled and doesn't want to be touched from behind without being asked first and waiting for a response.*

- *One person would only be in the bathroom alone with the door closed, while another had to have people with her all the time including using the toilet.*

- *Another didn't want people talking about her as if she wasn't there. She insisted that they use her name and not call her 'dear' or 'honey' or 'mom'.*

- *Another was concerned that breastfeeding would bring up neg-ative associations with a past experience involving their breasts. This person needed assistance in being anchored in the present whenever the baby nursed in those first few weeks.*

- *Others don't care for particular words, such as being told to 'relax'.*

This is the kind of information we really want to know as birth and postpartum doulas. How those needs came to be is not important. We don't need to know the story in order to be effective.

At this point your client may choose to tell you the story. But I think it's important to repeat that you don't need to know their story to help them. Disclosure should serve a purpose and you want to make sure they don't feel uncomfortable later if they tell you now. It could be a good time to get a glass of water or use the restroom to make sure their choice to disclose is one they've taken a few moments to consider. It is also okay for the doula to not want to know the story! Doulaing is a relationship and you get to take care of yourself too. Perhaps hearing their abuse or assault story would be triggering or upsetting for you. It might also make it harder for you to be their doula because you are now upset by what you heard (this is called secondary trauma). It is okay to ask that they keep their disclosure minimal or very general rather than including details.

My second point is that childhood sexual abuse is estimated to affect one out of every four women [1] in the United States, and one out of six men[2]. Sexual assault and rape are also common experiences[3], directly affecting at least twenty percent of the population. So, we're probably better off as doulas if we assume an assault or abuse history rather than seeing it as exceptional. That doesn't mean that every person who has been assaulted or abused will be affected by it during labor or their postpartum. In fact, some people are relieved to find that it didn't have a negative effect in that part of their life.

In my experience there are two behaviors that new doulas are most likely to see and that they can effectively address. The first is disassociation – for some reason, the person in labor or postpartum doesn't seem to be present anymore. They seem to be out of touch with what is happening with their body, their present moment consciousness is somewhere else. The person may seem distant and unfocused, or may even be looking out the window or down and to the left (recalling a memory). The empathetic neurons in the doula's gut are giving the message that the client isn't with you anymore in the room; they've drifted somewhere else.

For some people disassociation is an effective way of coping. Make sure you give your client the option of returning to the present moment and support them in their choice. "I notice that you don't seem to be present with us right now. Do you want me to help you be here with us or are you in a safe place in your mind?" If your client is safe, let them be. If family is there, they know the laboring person best and may be better able to support them.

Another worrisome situation is when the laboring or postpartum person's behavior seems to be totally out of proportion to what precipitated it. In other words, the way they are acting seems to be more dramatic or over the top and is disconnected from what they are responding to. This overreacting may mean they were reminded of something awful that happened in the past. They are responding to that experience rather that what is currently going on.

In both instances, the most effective actions are the same for a client who wishes to return to the present moment. Bring them back to the room with you, allowing the client to set the pace, and anchoring them in their senses. This generally works best when the doula is quietly and gently persistent, rather than using a loud voice or giving orders.

- Use your client's name, use today's date – or better yet, ask them what day and year it is.

- Have them look at you, have your client tell you what is happening today, and where they are.

- Have them notice objects in the room, prompting them with positive ones (flowers, baby book, etc.).

- If invited, touch them in a preferred way (you'll know them) in a safe place on their body (this will differ). If you aren't sure, *ask.* "May I put my hand on your knee, arm, hand?"

- Rather than ordering them to do something, invite them. Let the client choose – *this is very important.* "If you can, let yourself bring your attention to TODAY fully." "When you are ready, let yourself explore feeling safe here in the room with us, letting your body to birth/breastfeed/nurture your baby."

- When it seems that your client is mostly back in the present moment, ask something like, "How can I help you to feel more safe right now? Even if it seems silly, please tell me. Our brains sometimes have wisdom that doesn't make sense at first."

- Follow through as best you can, with the extra blanket or the pink flowers from the gift shop or finding the right song on the playlist.

These can seem to be scary situations for newer doulas, but we can use the same skills with our friends and family members who have experienced trauma and are triggered by something. Sometimes they aren't even aware that it happened, and our feedback is what helps them to notice that they aren't in the present moment anymore. To me, because so many people have experienced personal violation, these are life skills we all need to see one another through the journey. It's not about complicated strategies. It's about being a safe and trustworthy person and allowing the laboring or postpartum person to have their own experience in a supportive atmosphere.

Some doulas have extensive counseling skills, degrees, or training. They have additional strategies to use than what I've mentioned here. The book, *When Survivors Give Birth* by Phyllis Klaus and Penny Simkin, is an excellent resource. There are also facilitators offering two and three day comprehensive workshops for birth professionals wanting to focus on this issue in their practices.

[1] http://www.oneinfourusa.org/statistics.php

[2] https://1in6.org/the-1-in-6-statistic/

[3] http://centerforfamilyjustice.org/community-education/statistics/

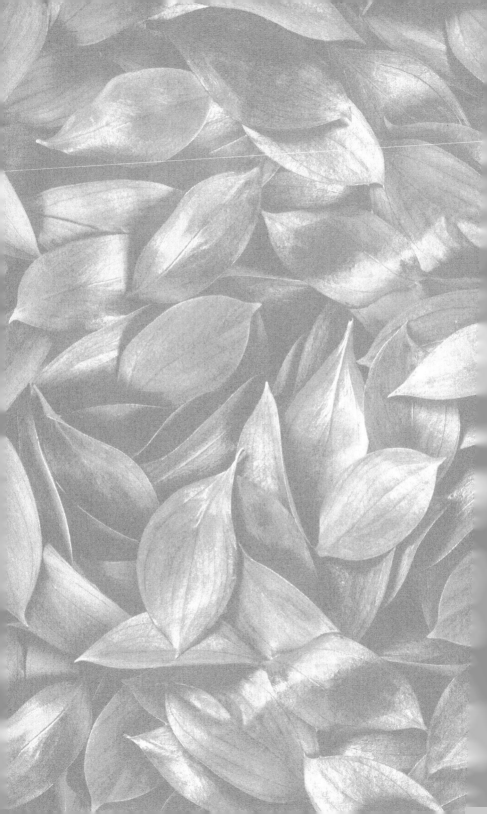

Medical
Professionals

Doulas: Why You Need
To Be Nice First

A doula was complaining on Facebook in response to one of my posts about getting along with nurses. *"Why do I have to be the one to put forth the effort? I wish some nurse would try to get along with me first."* According to the doulas in my study, here is why it's up to the professional birth doula:

- You are a guest in her house.

- Making the first move sets the tone for every communication and interaction that follows. Why not use this opportunity to your advantage?

- You only get one chance to make a first impression - and it takes three times as much experience with you to change someone's mind. Make those first minutes count.

- You are an ambassador for all birth doulas. Your actions reflect on all of us.

- Social skills and emotional intelligence are a significant part of a doula's success.

- "Hostess" is implied in our job description.

- Hospitals are set up for the mass production of a number of patients moving through the system. When you ask the nurse to change what she usually does to personalize care for your client (even when it is evidence based), she may get flak from other nurses or doctors for doing so. Therefore you need to be grateful when you hear "yes" and accept "no" graciously. (It doesn't mean your clients stop trying – it means you are polite.)

- The last doula may not have behaved optimally.

- As unfortunate as this is, a client may be treated negatively by the nurse or medical care provider because of their poorly behaving doula. I think we can all agree it is unacceptable to stress out anyone at a birth over our behavior.

- When you make an effort, especially a big one, the "norm of reciprocity" states the nurse will naturally want to keep things in balance. So you get what you give.

Doulas And Informed Consent

O ne of our primary functions is to empower the mother and her partner to ask questions. Many of us feel that a nudging, "Do you have any questions about that?" should get our clients more information in the labor room. Often I can tell them what they need to know, but I don't consider that to be my role. It also defeats one of my main unstated purposes: to increase communication and trust between patient and medical care provider (MCP). The more I assist information to flow from the doctor, nurse or midwife towards my client, the more improved their relationship will be. The laboring person and partner or family member can also evaluate their MCP and whether their approaches match. If I do the talking, those important processes don't take place. I know what I know so I can tell whether they are getting the information they need.

What if the laboring person and family aren't getting the information they need? What if an important piece is missing? Then I ask. Depending on the situation, a direct or indirect approach may be best.

Direct approach: "Is timing an issue with this procedure? Some other physicians at this hospital had mentioned that to me before?" I recommend never mentioning that you read something somewhere – it can be interpreted that you are trying to one up the MCP – bad move! But stating that you heard it from another MCP with equal status or that you observed it at another hospital works better. The direct approach works best when you *sincerely act curious.* You need to be really present with the thought – "Why is it being recommended this way?"

If you have another agenda or predominant emotion, especially a negative one, it is likely that your subliminal behavior will reveal that and be interpreted negatively– often on an unconscious level. Also be aware that your client also gets the message from your question that there are different approaches – which the MCP may not care for.

The indirect approach can also be referred to as the "Dumb Doula" approach. "Isn't there something about…um, well…the timing, is it called, with this procedure?" You are asking a leading question in a non-threatening voice. This strategy is designed to solicit information from the nurse, physician or midwife without challenging them or their authority. To be honest, I use this approach most often. It's been the most effective at meeting my client's needs over the years. Now the Dumb Doula approach is not without controversy. It certainly doesn't add to our professional reputation or appeal! "Those doulas might know how to rub a back, but you'd think they'd have learned some more technical stuff by now." Additionally, some doulas may think it is manipulative, that we aren't being authentic. To me, crafting communication strategies to maximize effectiveness is what I do all over my life: with my family, my students, and in mentoring situations.

Some physicians and midwives are happy to answer questions until their patients are comfortable with the recommended treatment or another decision has been reached. Others seem to feel that asking questions is equal to challenging their authority. They may seem brusque or annoyed. Often it is a clash of health care philosophies. Most people who have a doula want to be treated as individuals and to cooperatively make decisions with the doctor or midwife (who is probably a stranger). A MCP may see themselves as the knowledgeable authority whose role it is to make medical decisions. In addition, they will have to answer not only to the patient, but their colleagues, hospital administrators, their liability insurance company, and maybe a judge and jury. So doing what your client wants, rather their usual practice, can be a loaded proposition for a physician or midwife.

Having said that, doulas prompting clients to ask questions and receive answers actually helps the informed consent process. When mothers and their partners receive more complete information regarding procedures and intervention, this actually helps the MCP if an action is called into question. Why? Because the physician AND the nurse are supposed to separately chart every conversation with the patient[1]. The more discussion that is charted, the better that looks for the physician if there is a chart review for legal reasons[2]. Obstetricians who have been sued state that in retrospect, "they would spend more time with the patient and family" and/or "been more careful in the way I phrased things" and had "better chart documentation"[3]. These are areas where the doula's communication facilitation skills have the potential to help both the patient and the physician to receive and provide the best medical care possible. We already know that involved decision making and more complete information from MCPs leads to greater satisfaction for patients, and satisfied people are less likely to pursue a legal action.

When doulas help clients to get more information the result is a win/win for physicians and their patients. The more a laboring person knows before an intervention is done, the more satisfied they can be afterward – both immediately and weeks and months afterward. I just wish more physicians and nurses understood that.

---

1   Wisconsin Association for Perinatal Care Conference, 2016, *Document Like You'll Appear In Court, Hope You Never Will* by Jennifer Hennessy, JD, Quarles and Brady

2   ibid

3   Medscape Malpractice Report 2017: Why Ob/Gyns Get Sued by Carol Peckham https://www.medscape.com/slideshow/2017-obgyn-malpractice-report-6009316#20

The Doulas Have Arrived! Nurses, What Does This Mean For You?

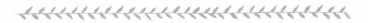

Dear Nurse,

When doulas move into a new area, nurses are often skeptical and hesitant to work with them. This is a normal reaction to change especially when you are uncertain about how it is going to affect you – and how you do your job. Here is a list written by an experienced doula trainer that might be helpful:

1. Professional doulas want to work *with you* to help a laboring person's needs get met. They view you as an important ally who has some of the same objectives and priorities.

2. The doula's goal is to remind their client to tell you and the physician or midwife what is most important to them about their birth. They may have listed their preferences on a one page birth plan or may only state them verbally.

3. Professional doulas do not have any agenda for a "natural" birth. Every person benefits from doula support - even people planning an epidural or cesarean section. They and their family benefit from the added nurturing, reminders they can discuss options, and extra hands that a professional doula can provide. A doula birth is a supported birth.

4. Professional doulas are familiar with the research evidence and best practices for maternal and fetal health. Many doula clients tend to also be familiar with this information – which is why they

hire a doula. Because of this, patients with a doula may make more requests than a less informed patient would. Some of these requests may already be allowed for in hospital protocols, even though the obstetrical unit's culture does not usually promote them. Some examples:

- No routine amniotomy

- Intermittent fetal monitoring

- Freedom to choose second stage positions outside of bed

- Hands and knees, kneeling and semi-sitting positions with an epidural

- Request a peanut ball

- Delayed cord clamping

- Baby's naked body on the birthing person's naked body immediately after birth and not removing it for 90 minutes or more (skin to skin)

- Delaying routine newborn procedures (but not health assessments) for 90 minutes or more

- Newborn exam on birthing person's body or their bed

- Weighing and bathing of baby in the patient's room

5. Patients who prefer a cooperative decision making relationship with their care provider often hire a doula to remind them to ask questions about their care. This interaction style may be rare in some obstetrical settings but is common in others. Rather than having their physician making all decisions, these patients expect

to be consulted and give explicit consent for each intervention. With these patients, the doula may ask if the birthing person and their partner have any questions about a proposed intervention. The ensuing discussion about benefits, risks, and options may be seen as an interruption or delay. However, involvement with decision making has been shown to increase patient satisfaction, birth satisfaction, and lower anxiety, lessen the incidence of post-partum depression and prevent post traumatic stress disorder due to a traumatic birth. Involvement in decision making has been repeatedly shown in the nursing literature to be more important than complications, length of labor, or location of birth to short and long term maternal well being.[4][5]

6. In order to facilitate involvement in decision making, a doula may tell the patient about an unannounced intervention the physician is about to do. This way the mother may give explicit consent or ask for clarification. The nurse or physician may see this as an interruption but this is what a doula accompanied patient expects their doula to do.

7. Despite these interruptions in the usual flow of care, the professional birth doula is your ally. They know the patient and can help you to get to know them more quickly. They will observe almost every contraction and can keep you informed of any concerns the laboring person has or adverse symptoms shy people may keep to themselves. Doulas help people in labor to stay focused.

---

4   Meyer, S. (2013). Control in Childbirth: a concept analysis and synthesis. *Journal of Advanced Nursing, 69*(1), 218-228.

5   Attanasio, L. B., McPherson, M. E., & Kozhimannil, K. B. (2014). Positive Childbirth Experiences in US Hospitals: A Mixed Methods Analysis. *Maternal and Child Health Journal, 18*(5), 1280-1290. doi:10.1007/s10995-013-1363-1

8. With a 60-80% epidural rate in most hospitals, some nurses do not see many unmedicated labors. Doulas have been trained in normal physiologic birth, as defined by the American College of Nurse Midwives (ACNM). Laboring people without pain medication may become louder and listen to their bodies' urges to move as labor intensifies. When people are coping well they are calm between contractions. The doula will help them to continue their coping ritual – which may become louder and more intense as labor progresses.

Three Clinical Recommendations:

When you are introduced to the doula, ask about their training and experience. Professional doulas are usually excited to tell you about their organization and background. If they have not taken training, then this person is the client's friend who is intending to doula them. But their friend is not a professional, so none of the descriptions in this essay apply. The "doula" friend may act in ways that a professional would not do, such as speaking for the person in labor, touching you or the physician inappropriately, arguing with you, giving medical advice or telling the person in labor what to do. These are NOT in the scope of practice of a professional doula. If they are doing these things and have been trained, this person is considered a *rogue doula*, behaving outside the circle of professional practice and ruining our reputation. We hope they go away even more than you do.

New doulas may make beginner mistakes. There are more new doulas than experienced ones. This is a challenging profession and many promising new doulas find it is not a good lifestyle fit. Please be patient with the beginning doula and help them learn how to treat you. They want to do their best to get along with you while helping their client to have the best birth possible. They may ask many questions about procedures and provider preferences until they become familiar with your facility.

Labor and birth are changing due to the doula's influence. But this is not necessarily a bad thing. Nurses are learning alternative approaches in non-pharmacological pain management and positioning techniques to rotate malpositioned babies. They are relearning the satisfaction of emotional connection to a patient that the doula helps to facilitate. They are seeing normal physiologic birth happen in their facility (even though it may require suspension or delay of usual interventions). But most of all, because of nurses and doulas working together, persons and babies are having emotionally healthy outcomes as well as physically healthy ones.

How Not To Be *THAT DOULA* In A Nurses' Mind

THAT Doula is the one the nurses roll their eyes at and don't want to see in the labor room. The one they aren't certain about, the one who leaves them wondering how their patient may be negatively influenced, the one they feel oversteps boundaries and has their own agenda – not the patient's - in mind. I've done extensive research interviews with doulas and nurses, consulted with nursing unit directors and served as a mentor doula. To me, the vast majority of the time these concerns arise from misunderstandings and miscommunication between doulas and nurses.

When we arrive at the hospital how do we counter the negative perceptions that nurses may have about a doula? (This is much harder when the hospital staff has had experiences with a rogue doula who behaves in these ways on a regular basis. That may require a more direct approach.) What I am talking about here is building your own reputation as a trustworthy doula. Often we can't do anything about the past, we can only begin with the next birth. Here are best practices culled from experienced doulas and labor and delivery nurses:

1. Smile. Smile when you meet someone, smile when they walk into the room, smile when you walk down the hall. Be genuinely you, don't fake smile. A person's brain perceives a smile as welcoming and automatically changes their behavior to be more receptive towards the person smiling at them. This is unconscious. So shifting your behavior to be welcoming by authentically smiling can use this tendency to your advantage.

2. Adjust your nonverbal behavior to be welcoming and acknowledge the MCP's presence when they come into the room or closer to the laboring mother's personal space. A head nod, slight shift in your shoulders or body orientation can indicate your awareness of their presence. You can do this while not taking your attention away from the person in their laboring, or wait until the contraction passes if needed.

3. Introduce yourself, share a little bit about yourself and what you are there to do. "Hi, Jordan. My name is Amy, I've been a doula for 20 years off and on. I'm here with Jamie and Shawn to help them with comfort measures, remind her to change positions, fetch things, and to remind Shawn to speak to you and Dr. X about what is most important about their birth."

4. If needed, explain what you do not do. "I don't do vaginal exams or anything clinical. I don't speak for Jamie and Shawn, I just remind them when it's a good time to mention their wants and needs with you or the doctor and midwife."

5. "Wonder with" and include the nurses when they are present. "I wonder if we might try…" "Shawn seems to be tiring, maybe a position change would be good??? What are you thinking?" "Are you noticing Shawn's contractions slow down when their mother is in the room or is it just me?" Nurses have been to hundreds of labors and may know coping strategies that we've never thought of. It is a courtesy to ask – remembering the laboring person is the decider.

6. Include the nurse in the laboring person's coping ritual whenever you can. Any connection you can enhance between them is good for their relationship. It also helps the person in labor to feel safer

and cared for. Nurses like to provide comfort measures but their other responsibilities limit their time.

7. Acknowledge the nurse's rank and her territory. If you are thinking about a big change, such as laboring in the tub or walking the unit, find the nurse and ask her before you do it. You might want to consider asking in a general way an hour or two before you make your move. "Shawn wanted to try laboring in the tub today. Is there any reason we ought to check with you first before doing that?" Some nurses don't need this communication, while others feel put out when their patient is doing something unexpected. There's nothing like going into a patient's room and finding them not there! If the physician calls and the nurse is out of the loop, the nurse looks less competent.

8. Do simple things that make the nurse's job easier. Pick up the dirty laundry, offer to get something to drink when going to the kitchen. Imagine yourself working together on the same team and building a relationship. You are! You are both on this mother's birth team along with her family members.

9. Urge the laboring person to speak up verbally about what they want to *each nurse and MCP*. "I really want to avoid an epidural" or "I want an epidural but Amy is going to help me to use the tub first to see if I like it." "Don't tell me to 'push, push'." Get the laboring person and their partner used to speaking up. Get their voice in early and often.

10. Prompt your client to speak up: "Shawn, do you want to tell the resident about your approach to pain medication?" Maybe a slower, gentler approach is better: "Hmmm, Shawn, I'm wondering if you want to share what's important to you with Dr. Y since

she's going to be involved with your care." You want your voice to be remembered as the one who is reminding the client, not the one who is saying the words for them.

11. If you've done the prompting and your client doesn't say anything, let it go. It is *their birth* and if their vision is not happening because they aren't saying anything then you have to let it go. A good general guideline: "I'll stick my neck out as far as my client does, but I won't go any farther.

12. "When a medical decision needs to be made invite the nurse to stay in the room." Since Jamie and Shawn have some time to discuss what to do next, Jordan, do you want to stay in case they have any questions?" By inviting the nurse to stay you avoid the appearance of being manipulative or unduly influencing your clients toward other approaches than the one being initially recommended.

13. Don't give medical information. Help your client to solicit that information from the medical staff. You know what you know so that you can tell if they are getting the information they need to make a good decision. You don't know it so that you can say it out loud to your client. The doula's role is to enhance connection and communication, not be the source of medical information. It is okay to ask leading questions *only if* your client has indicated she wants more information but it doesn't seem to be forthcoming. "Isn't there some kind of number or score about her cervix to consider when breaking her bag? I think Nora and I were talking about that a while ago."

14. Know what you know and don't claim to know what you don't know. If you are unfamiliar with position changes with an

epidural, say so. "I took a workshop where getting in a kneeling or hands and knees position with an epidural could help to prevent posterior positioning and labor dystocia. I haven't done it before, but Shawn would like to try it if possible. Do you think *we could work together* and see if that is good for Shawn and the baby?"

15. Realize that everyone present is providing what they feel is the best care for mother and baby. Almost all physicians, midwives and nurses are making the best recommendations possible based on their knowledge and experience while taking your client's preferences into account. It is the rare MCP who is misogynist or disregarding the emotional importance of childbirth. I'm not saying that it doesn't happen. I am saying that making that assumption *without direct experience* of it does a disservice to you, your clients, and the medical staff you are working with.

16. Repeat after me: "It's not your birth. It's not your birth. It's not your birth." Tattoo this in your memory, embroider it on the inside of your birth bag. It's not your birth! Our role is to follow the laboring person's lead even if it seems they're doing the opposite of what they said they wanted prior to labor. Don't have your own agenda for this birth or this person. Their birth is their life experience. Don't cheat them out of it just because we want it to be a different way. Our job is to support the choices a person is making now even when she may not stand up for herself or what she said she wanted earlier.

17. Your reputation precedes you and nurses will talk about you after you leave (perhaps even while you are there). Make sure that this nurse has good things to say about you – or at least nothing specifically bad. It may take more than one birth for positive feedback about you to circulate but it's worth it. Hopefully you

will experience greater satisfaction in your relationships with medical staff by following these strategies too.

18. Nurses have personalities, struggles with coworkers, worries, and families waiting for them. In other words, they are whole people. Show respect for them and concern for their needs. An approach that works with Nurse Jordan won't work with Nurse Terry. A large factor in your success as a doula is your ability to pay attention to other's cues and adapt your behavior to get along successfully with them. Our job is complex because we have to do this with our client, her family, her care providers and members of the nursing staff – simultaneously!!

These are advanced communication strategies that seem deceptively simple. It takes courage to change even when behaving in a way that is natural to us isn't getting the results we want. All of them are ways of being at a birth that highly effective doulas practice and that labor and delivery nurses said they appreciated. My hope is that they will help you find increased satisfaction and harmony in this critical aspect of doulaing.

How Professional Birth
Doulas Benefit Doctors

O ne of the neglected areas of research on doulas is their impact on physicians. Studies have shown that physicians have mixed feelings about the presence of birth doulas with younger obstetricians *of both genders* having the least positive attitudes (1). Commenting on this study, Klein stated:

> *"Perhaps most concerning, the obstetricians in the younger group were less favorable to birth plans, less likely to acknowledge the importance of the woman's role in her own birth experience, and more likely to view cesarean surgery as "just another way to have a baby".* (2)

Klein has also stated that there is diversity among the attitudes of both obstetricians and family physicians. At least 20% had attitudes similar to midwives and doulas regarding childbirth – especially experienced and older physicians. Even though our philosophies of birth may differ that does not mean that the presence of a doula is detrimental to physicians. In my estimation there are nine benefits that a professional doula can provide for physicians. In order of relevance, these include fostering informed consent, observing detailed progression of labor; assisting the physician to know the patient; providing continuous care and thus increasing patient satisfaction with the birth experience; fewer interventions; higher percentage of fees collected; informed refusal; early labor monitoring; and mitigating socially awkward situations.

Fostering informed consent. When the doula encourages the patient to ask their physician about an intervention, a common result is greater Information about risks, benefits, and alternatives. This enables the patient to make a more informed decision and give explicit consent for the procedure, which benefits the physician. It is no secret that obstetrical care providers are one of the most likely to be sued for malpractice (3). According to a physician conference presentation I attended in 2016 given by a malpractice attorney, any time discussion of a procedure can be documented it is positive for the physician. It strengthens the physician's position in case of a lawsuit even if it cannot protect him or her from its occurrence.

However, this discussion does not always fit smoothly into the course of a labor. As Morton explains, the doula can drive an "interactional wedge" between the patient and the physician (4). This occurs when the physician is preparing to conduct a procedure for which the laboring person has not explicitly given consent. As the doula has been trained to act and engaged by the client to do, they will inform the mother of the physician's actions before they are completed. ("It looks like Dr. X is preparing to break the bag of waters. Did you have any questions about that first?") The physician's activity is interrupted and they must interact with the patient about the procedure. If the doula were not there, this interaction would likely have proceeded without interruption or discussion between the patient and physician.

In the moment the medical care provider (MCP) may not be pleased with the doula or the interruption to what the MCP perceives as giving good care. It is possible the MCP perceives that there is no need for discussion or consent because it has already been given when signing the "consent for vaginal delivery" form. But there can be a difference between what a physician perceives as informed consent and what a patient perceives as informed consent. When the doula knows the patient's concerns, she or he is able to facilitate communication about topics where the patient wants more information and to be involved in decision making. However, this interaction can be awkward and resented by the physicians – even though it is ultimately to their benefit.

Getting to know the patient as an individual. The majority of the time in a busy hospital the attending physician has never met the mother. Even if a recent pregnancy appointment occurred, it is quite likely that the physician has seen dozens of women since this mother's last visit. When a doula is present, the medical care providers are urged to individualize their care for this patient. Doulas do this in subtle ways: we encourage laboring people and their partners to say what they want to their nurse, to remind the doctor of their priorities, and to write a brief birth plan for their hospital record. Our very presence is a huge reminder that these parents have thought about their birth and have taken action to see that their needs are met. Evidence suggests that both patients and physicians may be unprepared for these conversations or be uncertain how to proceed (1). In these instances the presence of a doula may be valuable to both.

When providers know the mother, they are able to shift their care in a way that aligns with this patient's priorities – while still acting in their comfort zone. The doula is also able to explain the physician's concerns in language familiar to the laboring mother. Without the doula, the physician has a harder time satisfying the needs of the patient and ensuring that their experience is a positive one. Once again, this depends on the physician's style. Medical doctors who like to treat all patients similarly may be irritated by requests to individualize care. MCP's who place a high priority on connecting with their patients will recognize how much easier that is when a doula is present.

Increasing patient satisfaction. Three of the most important factors influencing patient satisfaction during labor are the quality of the caregiver-patient relationship, involvement in decision making, and amount of support from caregivers (5). These factors are more influential than age, socioeconomic status, ethnicity, childbirth preparation, physical birth environment, perceived pain, immobility, medical interventions, and continuity of care. Patients who feel higher levels of satisfaction are less likely to sue (6). Several studies show that continuous support by a trained doula helps to increase overall satisfaction with the birth experience (7). When the doula increases communication with the physician, assists with informed consent for interventions, and provides effective labor support, mother's satisfaction with the birth is increased. The intervention of the doula may carryover into increased satisfaction with the physician and possibly fewer lawsuits.

Observing progression of labor. Undoubtedly, physicians and nurses see more labors and births than a professional doula. However, observation of those labors is intermittent. Doulas have the opportunity to be with women for the entire labor. We see the progression of labor more clearly and are attuned to subtle changes in the woman's behavior and contraction pattern. When a physician asks the doula about the mother's labor, the doula is able to report detailed changes. Physicians have reported that with my observations and their expertise, it is possible to forecast more accurately. MCP's may find this useful when making decisions about doing a cesarean on another patient, going to the clinic, or seeing their child's recital. Physicians often do not realize that the doula is a source of information about the patient that is beneficial to their decision making.

Lower intervention rates and healthier outcome. The most recent Cochrane Collaboration review of over 15,000 mothers in 22 studies confirmed that mothers with trained doulas are less likely to have certain interventions (7). Thus, the complications that may occur as a result of their use do not happen as often. Of course, the practice style of the physician and hospital policies are influential factors that have more impact than the doula's presence (7). However, for most laboring people the fewer interventions used, the healthier the outcomes are for both mother and child.

6. *Increased profit with a standard reimbursement rate*: Mothers who have doulas are less likely to use pharmacological methods of pain relief and receive fewer interventions (6). When the physician receives a pre-set reimbursement rate for a delivery, there may be more profit when fewer interventions are used (8,9). The same is true for hospitals that are billed and reimbursed separately from physician fees. This is only a benefit when charges are not itemized or the maximum reimbursement is more than the actual cost.

Informed refusal. When patients are uncooperative, the doula is sometimes blamed for their behavior. However, my research shows it is more likely that mothers and fathers with defensive attitudes hire doulas (10). Doulas are just not influential enough to change lifelong preferences about physicians or hospitals. (This also assumes that professional doulas are against hospital birth – which is not true.) Those patterns of behavior and beliefs are set long before doula services have begun. The professional doula's role is to support the birthing person in their decisions even if they are not what the physician or midwife would want. If the doula takes a neutral stance and is not trying to convince the patient to be compliant, the doula can be seen as part of the problem.

Informed refusal is a part of informed consent and the right of every patient. However, it sometimes appears that the patient is personally distrustful of the physician or that their actions show a lack of care for their child. Misunderstandings often occur because this is an emotionally charged event for both patient and doctor. Sometimes the doula is highly skilled at negotiating the communication so that both parties understand one another even though they disagree. No matter when it occurs, informed refusal is a risk for both doctor and patient.

The doctor is being asked to practice in a way that is less than preferred and the patient may experience a drop in the physician's good feelings towards them. The benefit for the physician to having a doula present is to facilitate communication and to realize there is a person close to the patient who can understand the physician's legitimate concerns.

Early labor observation and support. When the professional doula is at home with the laboring client, they are able to provide reassurance. Birthing people may choose to stay at home until active labor is established rather than arriving too early by hospital standards. With the new definition of active labor commencing at 6 centimeters, observing early labor becomes even more important. Because doulas do not check cervixes, our observational skills are more highly attuned to behavioral signs of advancing labor. The experienced doula may see overt signs of an impending delivery or emergency that family members may miss. The doula can recommend calling the triage center for advice or emergency services when imminent help is required. The doula's skilled observation provides an additional level of safety for the patient that may benefit the physician.

Mitigate socially awkward situations. Physicians are often required to get to know several patients in rapid succession. Labor often includes meeting and interacting with extended family. Not all patients or providers are socially skilled and some situations make it much harder for people to get along. While the doula, nurse, midwife and physician are all professionals; influences of family structure, language, culture, exhaustion, and personality converge to create a number of challenging and awkward social situations. When the doula knows the family and the client's desires, they can head off or smooth over awkward situations for the physician. Simply introducing everyone properly may defuse tension.

Relationships between doulas and physicians can be tricky. The doula's presence indicates a desire on the part of the patient to be involved in decision making and to receive individualized care. The doula is the only professional on the birth team who is not beholden to the physician or the hospital, but to the patient. However, this part of the doula's role – to increase communication, understanding, and respect between physician and patient is a benefit to the doctor. Doulas increase patient satisfaction rates in a multitude of ways, which is also a benefit to physicians. When doctors understand how professional doulas benefit them and learn to utilize their expertise, they can make the birth less stressful for everyone.

1. Klein, M.C., Liston, R., Fraser, W.D., Baradaran, N., Hearps, S. J., Tonkinson, J., Kaczorowsky, J., Brant, R. (2011) Attitudes of the New Generation of Canadian Obstetricians: How do they differ from their predecessors? *Birth* 38:129-139.

2. Klein, M.C. (2011) Many women and providers are unprepared for an evidence- based, educated conversation about birth. *J Perinat Edu* 20:185-187.

3. Jena, A.B., Seabury, S., Lakdawalla, D., Chandra, A. (2011) Malpractice Risk According to Physician Specialty *New Engl J Me*d 629-636

4. Morton, C., Clift, E. (2014) *Birth Ambassadors: Doulas And The Re-emergence Of Woman-Supported Birth In America* Praeclarus Press 2014; 4:210

5. Hodnett, E.D. (2002) Pain and women's satisfaction with the experience of childbirth: a systematic review. *Am J Obstet Gynecol* 186:S160-72

6. Stelfox, H.T., Gandhi, T.K., Orav, E.J., Gustafson M.L. (2005) The relation of patient satisfaction with complaints against physicians and malpractice lawsuits. *Am J Med*, 118:126-133.

7. Hodnett, E.D., Gates, S., Hofmeyr, G.J. & Sakala, C. (2013) Continuous support for women during childbirth. *Cochrane Database of Syst Rev*

8. Chapple, W., Gilliland, A.L., Li, D., Shier, E., Wright, E. (2013) An economic model of the benefits of professional doula labor support in Wisconsin births. *WMJ* 112:58-64.

9. Kozhimannil, K.B., Hardeman, R. R., Attanasio, L. B., Blauer-Peterson, C., O'Brien, M. (2013) Doula care, birth outcomes, and costs among Medicaid beneficiaries. *Am J Public Health* 103:e1-9

10. Gilliland, A.L. (1998) Nurses, doulas, and childbirth educators: Working together for common goals. *J Perinat Edu* 7:18-24.

11. American College of Obstetricians and Gynecologists. (2014) Safe prevention of the primary cesarean delivery. Obstetric Care Consensus No. 1. *Obstet. Gynecol.* 123: 693-711.

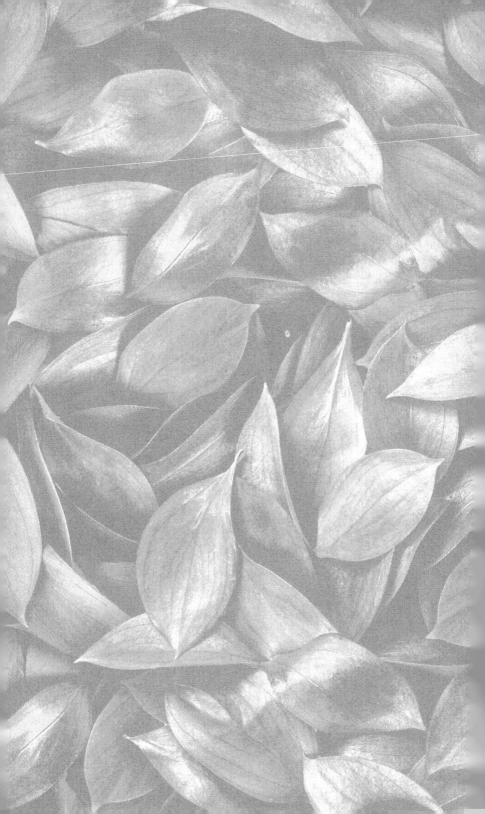

Powerful Prenatal Relationships

Powerful Prenatal Relationships

W hat most doulas want is to guide their clients to have memorable life experiences that contribute to positive parenting. We want our clients to be empowered and treated with respect; to know their options and choose wisely; to feel that our personal sacrifices were worth it for the difference we made in that family's life. Prenatal visits are the vehicle for arriving at that place, but most of us are uncertain how to go about consciously creating a supportive and professional relationship. We know it isn't the same as other healthcare relationships – there's more personal intimacy and less power difference than with medical care providers or mental health counselors.

This guide is based on my research with over forty doulas and thirty parents as well as my own experiences as an expert doula and doula trainer. I'll guide you through the more subtle nuances of building positive and impactful prenatal relationships. The key is to become a trustworthy and safe person. With that as your foundation, you can help another person transform into a better version of themselves simply through the power of your presence. That's the way lasting change happens.

Become A Safe Person

At the beginning of any relationship, trust is mingled with hope and uncertainty. Your client wants to trust you and offers one golden opportunity to prove yourself. If you flub it up, it will take three times the effort to get another one. However, you really don't want your clients to trust you automatically simply because you're their doula. Our goal is for them to trust themselves as decision makers. They've already decided to engage your services. Now they will look for evidence that it was a good choice. To prove that:

1.   Be reliable. Be on time. Do what you say you are going to do. Don't promise what you cannot deliver. If you aren't sure that your colleague has the book to lend, don't say you can get it. Say you will ask.

2.   Be organized. Know your calendar. Make sure your resources are in your bag or tablet and easily available.

3.   Be professional. Dress modestly to match their culture and climate – you don't want to be sexier than the pregnant person.

There are some caveats. Each one of these steps is easy to define but maybe not so easy to practice. While I can tell you to be organized or not to make false promises, these may be life changing challenges. Remember, it isn't required for you to be this way all over your life, just in your relationship with clients. Second, if you are doulaing cross-culturally norms for timeliness and dress may be different. Adapt to the customs that you know about and ask how to be more accommodating. Ask what you should know to help them best. My outlook is as an American White person, so these are the norms associated with competence in my culture, but they don't necessarily carry over to other social or ethnic groups. Listen to what I have to say with that in mind.

Make A Map Of Their World

Think of yourself as an explorer in new territory and be genuinely curious about what it means to be your client. I like to make a drawing of concentric rings – like a target. The outer rings are the influences of the outer world: birthing practices in your region, economy, majority culture values, and so forth. The next inner circle shows the influences of their community: friend's births, extended family values, religious group membership, health education, perinatal resources, etc. The next circle contains the people and events that directly affect them: physician/midwife availability, other children, past births, trusted others, stable housing, transportation issues, job security, etc. At the center are the birthing person and their intimate partner(s), their individual needs, personalities, and characteristics.

The better I can understand their world, the more effectively I can assist in coming up with possible solutions to problems. I can help others to relate to my client's worldview in a conflict. I know how to package information because I understand their stressors and perspectives. You don't have to use my model, but I find that drawing it on paper engages a creative part of my brain. The empathy neurons are activated. Putting the effort into mapping their world can increase your creativity and confidence in your problem solving ability.

4. Map their world. You'll be more effective at emotional support, pinpointing solutions and explaining the mysteries of perinatal care tailored to meet their individual needs.

Part of my personal history process is to collect the birth stories pregnant people have stored in their head. Some of those stories will take them where they want to go and some will keep them stuck. These deeply embedded memories influence our clients' beliefs about their own bodies and abilities to labor. When we can help them to unpack those often irrational ideas and shake them out, they lose their power. Sometimes this is the most constructive part of all my prenatal visits – getting to the heart of childhood fears or adult anxieties from their friend's experiences. It is also a rapport building strategy. "What stories did you grow up with about birth?"

It matters less what you say and matters more that you explore these stories for their hidden meanings and relevancy for this pregnancy and birth. Don't let them be put on the shelf unexamined. Sometimes partners carry scary birth stories that feed their anxieties during labor. When appropriate do this same exercise with them. They have a strong influence on labor progress, and their level of trust in the birth process makes a critical difference.

5. Keep a log of the influential birth stories that shaped your client's ideas about what labor and birth mean, what it will be like, and whether they are capable. When they come up in labor, you'll have a plan on how to address it.

Build Your Relationship Over Time

The most potent time for any relationship is its inception. You are getting familiar with one another, and as the doula you set the boundaries for the relationship. Make sure you let your clients know what types of communication work best, how and when to contact you, and how often. It is usually sufficient to write, "In the early months I usually hear from my clients every two weeks or after a prenatal appointment."

People who are emotionally needy or have multiple emotional challenges may begin to call or text you more often than you might want. But you can't put a limit on communicating *after* they've already started to contact you every day. If you try to dodge "too many" texts or calls, it can affect their confidence that you'll be available when they're in labor. If you are supporting cross-culturally, make sure you understand first what their expectations are of you. This is true even if you are a White person doulaing a Black family. American Whites aren't raised to think of ourselves as having a culture of our own or Black people as having a different culture, but that is the case. So just ask what their support needs are, how they want to communicate, and negotiate what will work for both of you. Once you know what to expect from one another, the relationship can grow authentically.

6. Set boundaries around your relationship with clients. Boundaries are not negative! They let everyone know what's expected so you can relax and build an authentic relationship. They reduce conflict and invite intimacy. Let your clients know expectations about payments, number of visits, scheduling, and how often you'll want to hear from them. Some people will need encouragement to contact you more often, while others will need to know not to text you every day.

As you spend more time together, it can feel natural to share personal stories and anecdotes about your life with your client. However, this is not a mutual friendship, this is a person who is engaging with you for a service. Even an innocuous story could take the conversation in unexpected directions. Be deliberate – think ahead of time about what you want to share and why. In general, keep it lighthearted.

The hard part comes when your client asks you a question about yourself and you aren't sure why. "Tell me about your births" is a common example. First you have to stop yourself from answering automatically like you would with a friend! Next, ask why they want to know. Maybe they want to get closer to you; maybe they're trying to figure out whether you've faced a similar dilemma. The trap is that pregnant people may compare themselves to you and then judge themselves negatively. This is easily avoided IF we take the time to ask and understand our client's needs first. (For more, please read *Why Not To Share Your Birth Story*.)

7. Share personal information only when it is the best strategy to meet your client's needs, but make sure you understand what the need is first.

Believe In Them Before They Believe In Themselves

As doulas, part of our role is to inspire. We need to trust deep down that birth works, that people's bodies can do what they were meant to do, and that people are capable of making important decisions about their lives and dealing with the consequences. Iris, a doula from Long Island, said, "I tell every single client, even somebody who's had a previous cesarean, I'm expecting things to unfold beautifully, exactly as they're meant to. That this is a very normal, very natural event unless your body tells us otherwise. And it's very rare that bodies do that without other things intervening."

One of the mothers in my study, Jessie, said early in her pregnancy she doubted she had any control over what happened. Then sometime after her second prenatal visit with her doula, things changed. She said it was like a switch inside of her turned on. "Like now, I know my pregnancy, like my pregnancy tells me something that the hospital does not, despite their good intentions that this is supposed to be done and this and this. If I didn't have those tests, I would probably trust that the pregnancy is good because I know what's going on." Jessie learned to trust her body and directly linked her doula's confidence in her to her own developing belief in herself.

8. Trust birth. Trust bodies. Belief comes across in the small things we say and do in each interaction. "I believe you will make the best decisions for yourself." "I believe you are capable of knowing what is right for you and your baby." While we might say those

things once or twice, it is how we act the rest of the time that makes a difference.

Create Opportunities For Empowerment

Doulas don't empower anybody; we create opportunities for people to empower themselves. We interrupt the procedure by asking, "Did you have any questions about that?" We teach BRAND or BRAIN acronyms for decision making. Our presence in the room means it is more likely that our clients will be involved with their care providers – even if we don't say or do anything. Our clients who are not used to having choices in their medical care or receive Medicaid may need more assistance in getting their voice heard than those who are in private pay systems. Amplify their voices by repeating what they said they wanted. Engage nurses in being a part of this client's labor and support that connection. We want everybody to be involved in creating the best birth possible as our client defines it. As several doulas in my study put it, "the mother's goals become my goals."

What else contributes to empowerment? Understanding your client's context of birth and reflecting that context back to them. For some people it is what you have to go through to get a baby. For others it is a journey of personal growth and spiritual development. For each of these clients the way you talk about labor and birth would be different, because you want your language and support strategies to fit into their paradigm.

Lastly, defuse the mysteries of labor and birth where you can. Forecast what to expect in the hospital, the range of available options, techniques for coping with sensations, and predicting potential conflicts and their resolution strategies.

9. Look for opportunities for your client's wishes or preferences to be known. Model asking questions in a way that shows others how your client prefers to be treated. Make sure clients speak up early and often. Enhance the connection between clients and care providers. Be kind.

Be Present With Your Heart And Your Head

Many of the practices to being a good doula are also ones that test our spirit. Patience. Acceptance. Allowing. Being present only in the moment. Listening. Trusting. These are what our clients need from us to flourish. Many of these principles have to do with who we are as people as well as the way we behave. We have to use our heads and our hearts when understanding our clients and their choices.

Joseph Chilton Pearce, a founder of the prenatal psychology movement, once told me, "The heart makes decisions, not the head. You need to understand that when working with parents." So, even when you give high quality evidence to people, they may still make choices that are puzzling. Your role is to trust them to make their own best decisions, especially when you don't know why. You don't need to understand another person's inner truth to support them. You only need to believe that they know what is best for them. That can be easier when you realize there is a greater principle at work.

Whether your clients see it this way or not, the perinatal period is transformative. At the end you are not the same person as when you started. Our role is to remember these deeper truths as we guide people. Even though individuals have their own journey, the terrain is knowable. It is familiar to us. It isn't scary. We help people let go of what was, even when they don't know what is coming next. We bridge that gap because they trust us.

10. Facilitate transformation by being present with your clients in your heart. Help them find their own truth and vision. Serve as a guide through the terrain of pregnancy, labor, birth, and postpartum. Normalize their experience. Translate the mysterious behaviors of people and procedures in their birthing facility so that clients understand them.

Know Yourself And Your Own Worth

Doulaing is work of the heart. Like therapists or counselors, what we do requires an authentic connection between the doula and the client. We see them at their most raw and vulnerable and do not shy away. Instead we move closer. It makes a difference that we started out as strangers. We co-created this relationship out of nothing so it could function for a specific and special time of transition. We are able to become whoever they need us to be. Then we allow our connection to dissipate until it is intermittent or nonexistent in the months and years after the birth.

Simultaneously, in our capitalist society people give us money for this service. We're expected to be business people and put a monetary price on our caring. What that means is that people have recognized that our service has value and meaning. When it becomes a commodity, something that can be bought and sold in the market, it is seen as valuable. The way we exchange what we have for what we want to acquire is by using money or barter. That's all money is – a system of energetic exchange using a common medium. It's not about your personal worth as a human being. You're commodifying your caring skills and they have a price. You deserve to be paid what you are worth. If others do not recognize that your skills have worth, that is a problem of perception. They don't understand the problems that having a professional doula solves.

11. Being a doula is a unique profession. We deal with the intangible and the unexplainable. We stand in our own strength letting things be the way they are without trying to fix them or pretty them up. We are deeply intimate during a vulnerable transition in people's lives. Then we move away, having helped them to find strength and abilities they didn't know they possessed. Our services are valuable and needed. When we hold this as truth inside ourselves, we know who we are. That transforms everybody.

My perspective on doulaing is unique. I've done the work, trained a thousand other people to do the work, and researched it for over fourteen years. I supported my first birth at twenty years old before I was a fully formed adult. In my own way, I'm immersed in the world of doulas! Having had so many prenatal relationships myself, I can state that these eleven principles have been refined over time. They work. Some of them are likely already familiar to you – they should be if you're a doula. But it is when you put them all together – your inner work on yourself and your approach to clients – that you will truly be able to have powerful transformative relationships that create lasting positive change in their lives.

Most people associate doulas and coping with labor. But the doula experience can be so much more: an experienced guide for a lengthy life transition that many of us are unprepared to make. Simply by being trustworthy, caring within boundaries, believing in and having a deep appreciation for our clients, we can help them transform into parents who believe in themselves and have confidence in their instincts. We leave them with so much more than they ever thought possible. None of this has to do with double hip squeezes, epidurals or birth outcomes.

It all begins and ends with who the doula is on the inside. That's where we have the most power to be transformative for anyone, especially ourselves.

Afterword

W hen I originally did this research analysis, ideas about race and the different identities doulas would bring to the doula-client relationship were not first on my mind. My goal was to distill the wisdom gleaned from the doulas in my sample. In 2017, I began interviewing birth doulas again. I was curious about what had changed but my listening was also different. In American culture our perspective of the world changed. Race is now part of many of our conversations; at least, it is now part of many of mine. Since 2014, when the first reports about racial disparities in birth outcomes became known in my community, I set out to change those statistics. The best place to do that was inside myself – after all White people, including White women, created this problem. It took about two years and a lot of race workshops before I was able to talk about race competently. It took another two years before I had a sense of my own White identity and could recognize whiteness in other people's behaviors.

In revising this book the last several rounds, I looked for information from my culture of Whiteness that isn't recognized as such. There are things that matter that doulas do that are "human being" things, like listening. It doesn't matter who you are, being listened to deeply is powerful for everyone. The vast majority of the solutions in this book are best practices for human beings. But then there are also suggestions that apply best for more privileged people, such as speaking directly to a physician and asking questions about what they are doing. This could backfire on our clients depending on the circumstances of the birth and the individual nature of the medical careprovider.

Depending on your culture and the cultures and worldviews of your clients and their caregivers, some suggestions in this book will be useful and some others may not. You will need to evaluate the suggestions in this book in light of what your clients consider to be kind and respectful behavior, and adapt your actions accordingly.

More than anything, I trust my readers. The individual doula will need to note when what is suggested does not work with your clientele, your or their culture, or the reality of their lives. I learned long ago in parent support meetings to "take what you like and leave the rest". Everyone reading this has innate wisdom based on their life experience. Let this book blend with what you know to be true and propel you forward to who you can be.

Acknowledgements

After working on this project for over a decade there are many people to thank. Most important are all the doulas who shared and reflected with me about the births they attended and people they supported. *The Heart of the Doula* reflects your hearts and your wisdom.

Ruth Ancheta has been my sounding board and main editor for over a decade now. Thank you Ruth for making my intentions clearer and better able to be heard. Katy Sticha, thank you for your administrative support and friendship. Without you I might never have turned a few blog posts into the book everyone is now reading. Over twenty five years ago Karen Kohls showed me birth through her eyes as a physical therapist. Thank you so much for all the other ways you've shown me the world, and your deep and abiding friendship.

Lastly, my children suffered through many grilled chicken breast dinners when I was collecting, analyzing, and writing up my data. Now you are all grown up making dinners in your own kitchens. Thank you for being my family and supporting me all the way through.